The
Berkowitz
Diet Switch

The Berkowitz Diet Switch

by

Gerald Berkowitz, M.D.

and

Paul Neimark

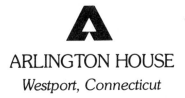

ARLINGTON HOUSE
Westport, Connecticut

To Debbie—
My wife, my lover, my friend.

G.B.

To Rick—
A genius who is also a genius
at being human.

P.N.

Library of Congress Cataloging in Publication Data

Berkowitz, Gerald.
    The Berkwitz diet switch.

    Includes index.
    1. Reducing diets. I. Neimark, Paul G.,
joint author. II. Title.
RM222.2.B453   613.2′5   80-26419
ISBN 0-87000-481-6

MANUFACTURED IN THE UNITED STATES OF AMERICA
1 2 3 4 5 6 7 8 9

Contents

PART ONE

Enjoyable Weight Control

1

Why This Diet Should Work Where All the Others Have Failed You

CORRECT ME IF I'M WRONG: YOU NOW ARE, OR IN the near future again will be, overweight.

You plan to embark upon a "diet," half hoping that some newly touted twist of something you've already tried will permanently prevent those extra pounds from returning. Yet, underneath, you know that you'll wind up in the same old take-it-off-put-it-on-take-it-off-put-it-on trap. But you'll probably try the diet anyway for three good reasons: (1) you'll look better, (2) you'll feel better, and (3) if the diet is safe and you don't go about it in an unsafe manner, you'll be healthier.

Because you—and virtually everyone else you've

known—have been hurt, however, by the vicious circle of the take-it-off-put-it-on pattern, you may go at it only halfheartedly and "fail" even sooner than before. Or you may accept your overweight. Or, knowing that all these past diets have failed you and future ones likely will as well, you may opt for what you think is the only other alternative: "willpower." Less than 1 percent of those who are overweight succeed with "willpower"—but *not* because of a lack of willpower. You have far more willpower than you might imagine, as do the overwhelming majority of people I've known. Please stop a moment and think how, each day, you cope countless times with a difficult, much too fast-paced, often hostile world, to say nothing of having to handle your own personal problems. No, willpower is not what you lack. What you "lack" is the knowledge of this crucial fact: *willpower has next to nothing to do with weight loss.*

What I want to tell you about is a simple, effective, permanent weight-loss technique that requires little or no willpower. To begin with, I want to answer the key question you no doubt already want to ask—the same question I had to ask myself time and again during my research and testing: *What makes the Berkowitz Diet Switch different?*

The answer is that, first, *The Berkowitz Diet Switch is not a diet.* It is *the* diet. In one sense, it is *every* safe diet you have ever tried.

You see, there are less than a dozen basic types of diets. Every reducing regimen you've ever been on is a variation on one of them. And all of them work, for awhile, *not because of what they are, but simply because you're on a diet. Their temporary "success" stems almost solely from the fact that they are a diet, from the fact that you are dieting again.* The proof of this pudding is that some of the most popular are what I call the Gimmick Diets, that is, there is absolutely no solid physiological or medical evidence as to why they work.One popular weight-reducing plan of the 1970s, for example, did not claim to know why the diet worked. But the author had tried it, she said, her friends had tried it, and it worked. So millions of Americans tried it.

Unfortunately, the temporary success of the Gimmick Diet—and all the other types of diets—*is inextricably fused with their inevitable failure.* My six-and-a-half year sampling of a wide cross section of people who tried the eight diet types yields the following figures:

After	% Still On That Diet
1/4 year	67
1/2 year	48
1 year	26
2 years	13
3 years	6
6 years	3

Why do these diets fail us (and *they* fail *us, we don't* fail *them*) so quickly and, after awhile, so completely? They fail because their two positive ingredients are "eaten up" faster than circus cotton candy. One ingredient is their newness— the excitement and hopefulness surrounding them. Obviously, that can't last very long. The second is their support, their results, since in the beginning you'll lose weight on almost any diet. But when, after you've lost that first 15 (or even 50) pounds and start struggling, struggling, *struggling* for the next five pounds, two, one, then begin gaining, the support is zero.

So, too soon, the diet that made you so happy, that you praised to your family and friends, becomes a constant demand, an unrelenting pressure, In a word, it turns into your worst enemy!

The Berkowitz Diet Switch (BDS) differs from all the diets that have failed you *because the newness and the support are permanent.*

How is this accomplished?

By your switching from diet to diet to diet.

Let's say you're 38 pounds overweight. You answer ten simple questions. Your answers tell you which BDS diet to begin with, which to switch to next, and what switches to make after that.

So, you begin on a diet tailored to *you,* not an unnatural weight-reducing method that you fall into at random because it's popular or is temporarily working for someone you know.

With the BDS, you succeed on each diet, and get out while the getting is still good.

You answer a second handful of simple questions, and switch to a second diet. And, within a brief period of time, lose from 5 to 9 pounds.

And switch.

And lose from 3 to 5 pounds.

And switch.

And, for a short duration, merely maintain your weight loss.

And switch again.

And lose.

And switch once again.

And attain your ideal weight.

Too simple? For *you*, it will be very simple. For me, it required years of research that was so painstaking it made medical school seem like a Sunday afternoon in front of the TV set.

It was worth it, however, because not only did I discover that you can achieve your ideal weight for good, but that something even more important takes place in the process, the most important thing of all:

ENJOYABLE, WEIGHT-CONTROLLING EATING HAS BECOME
A WAY OF LIFE TO YOU.

While you have been switching, losing pounds, keeping pounds off, the Berkowitz Diet Switch has replaced not only the unsuccessful reducing plans that failed you, but *has replaced your own eating lifestyle that resulted in over-weight.*

In a word, the switching of diets has become *the* diet. For the first time, and for good, an enjoyable way of eating has become a permanent part of your life.

And *enjoyable* is the key word.

Probably the most frequent complaint I encountered from dieters over eight years was that the dieting dominated their lives. "Even while my reducing plan was working," one woman expressed it, "it wasn't worth it. Because most of the time all I could think about was eating—or *not* eating.

When could I eat next? Should I eat this? How much of that? Had I overeaten? Had I stuck to the diet? Food became by far the most important part of my life. And the worst of it was that I wasn't enjoying it as much as before I went on the diet."

Why is *the enjoyment of eating* such an important facet of the Berkowitz Diet Switch?

The unhappy eater is, ultimately, the overeater. All of the various diets I've ever seen, to a greater or lesser degree, treat your appetite, your love of food, your body, *you,* like a naughty child or a rank animal. Some will let you eat some of what you want, sometimes big portions of it. Yet didn't you have the feeling that someone was standing over you with a club? The longer you stayed on the diet, the more apprehensive you became that the ax was about to fall, since the only way you could hope to keep shedding pounds was to pound away at that same menu month after month.

Well, in a sense your body is a child. And a child, if treated right, will treat you nicely in return.

Make it happy. Feed it.

The Berkowitz Diet Switch encourages this, and by satisfying probably your most important sensory need (because food is not only taste, but touch and sight and smell as you take it into your mouth and swallow), you usually release yourself from thinking about food and dieting until just before the next time you eat. People on the BDS find that they enjoy food more, but think about it less.

Yet the BDS goes past even this, which is one of the things that makes it unique. *It selectively* encourages you to *overeat.*

Because you will, you know. Virtually everyone does. So

this factor is built *into* your eating plans. Soon you'll find you're *planning* your overeating! And, if you don't plan it yourself, you'll find yourself doing it anyway. Depending on what stage you're at in the BDS, you're allowed from three to five overeatings weekly. They will not ruin your diet, they will not throw you off your diet. It is *part* of your diet.

Contrast this with any other "diet." Break it for a day, and you feel the diet is destroyed. And much of your self-esteem with it.

The BDS employs proven metabolic principles, but physiologically and psychologically positive ones. Moreover, the order of the diets as you switch is based upon solid behavioral principles. This is one reason why you lose those next 9 or 10, then 5 or 3 pounds after your first 19 or 25 as you make your several switches. And, not incidentally, several switches within each cycle are all you may make, because one or two Diet Types may *not* be for you.

And I think the chances are huge that you will find the four or five or half-dozen eating plans on your Berkowitz Diet Switch a treat, not a treatment.

People seem to find each facet of the BDS an adventure, and the prospect of each new switch a singular incentive. Gone is the physically unhealthy, emotionally enervating "double message" of the gain and lose, gain and lose, gain and lose cycle. Gone is guilt—that unfair and, for many people at times, unbearable feeling of having "failed" again where it was impossible in any case to succeed. Gone is the all-encompassing limbo of really not knowing what to do next.

Most of all, *gone are the pounds.*

2

I Discovered Diet-switching Because of My Own Overweight

I'M AMAZED AT THE NUMBER OF PEOPLE WHO HAVE given their hard-earned money to stockbrokers to invest without inquiring whether the brokers have made real money themselves that way. Or the couples who see marriage counselors whose own marriage has broken up or is floundering.

If you take the advice of a supposed expert on something, he or she would be expert for one reason and one reason only: he's done it himself. There is too much "experting" today by people who have merely studied their subject rather than truly mastered it. Would it make sense for the Pittsburgh Steelers to start a quarterback who had never completed a pass but had studied football assiduously for ten years?

And there seems to be more secondhand experting in the field of reducing than almost any other. I always think of the doctor I saw on TV some years ago who had become a leading diet expert. Just a glance at him would tell you—as it told me—that he had one of those body types that never get fat. Was he a good ad for his diet—or for having lean parents and grandparents?

I found diet-switching because I was fat, wanted to lose weight, and hadn't been able to do it on any of the "tried and true" reducing plans. When I was first married, I weighed 170 pounds. Slowly over the next few years I accumulated weight, not really being aware of it, as my practice thrived and I settled into a more sedentary existence. When I entered the Air Force four years after I got married, I was sent to a relatively isolated base in the upper peninsula of Michigan with my family. My weight continued to balloon. After a year and a half I weighed over 210 pounds and looked every ounce of it. For the first time, friends and family who saw me at three- to four-month intervals began to comment that I indeed looked "fat." What a surprise to one who weighed 155 pounds at a little over six feet at the age of twenty-four—and used to worry on the beach because my ribs showed!

Then, unexpectedly, a sudden change occurred in my lifestyle. My wife began to feel very tired and rapidly lost energy. One evening I noticed she had turned yellow! Tests soon confirmed a rather severe case of hepatitis, requiring hospitalization and then long-term convalescence with her family in Chicago. I was suddenly left adrift in a situation to which I was unaccustomed. After five years as a pampered husband, I found myself too lazy to relearn preparing my own meals. So I took the easy way out. I began eating less of everything, feeling that it wouldn't hurt me, since I was overweight anyway. With the help of a friendly chef at the base hospital, I began a high-protein, low-carbohydrate diet and stopped eating snacks at home. Since I didn't care for fish and seafood, my meals were somewhat limited in scope, but ultimately I succeeded in losing close to 20 pounds in just over a month.

Needless to say, in time I became monumentally bored with the diet and went off it with a bang—stocking up my house with all kinds of snacks and driving off base to all the fast food outlets and easy-to-eat foods. Within several weeks I was up to almost 210 pounds again—and feeling very lonely and frustrated at my inability to cope.

It was then I realized for the first time that what I should have done when I tired of the high-protein, low-carbohydrate diet was make a diet *switch*. Instead of going off the diet and stuffing myself with useless calories, I should have switched to another diet to maintain an effective but different reducing method.

Upon seeing this, I first returned to my original diet, and within weeks was down to 195 pounds. When I got tired and bored with that diet, I *switched*. A little over a month later, I switched again. And I kept switching, sometimes returning to my original diet, sometimes moving on to a new diet. Soon I was back in the 170s.

How did I know which diets to switch to? I *didn't* know, at least not nearly as much as I do today. It wasn't until years later that I began testing my method seriously on others and perfecting it. However, I did apply my medical knowledge and the studies I had made of nutritional needs, so even then the diets I devised were a healthy progression, and, as important, never became boring. In fact, the idea of sensibly switching diets became so fascinating to me that it became my avocation more or less, and still is.

I became so excited over my success that I began utilizing it on some of the patients I would see in the infirmary. Unfortunately, they were usually poorly motivated, did not keep appointments for follow-up, and were frequently transferred. The civilian patients were mostly older dependents or retired personnel not interested in dieting. Even then, some of the results were dramatic. But I decided to wait for a full-scale test until I was in private practice.

As I said, I had gotten my weight down to less than 180 pounds. Meantime, my wife had recovered fully. Home-cooked meals were prescribed to help her regain her weight-loss. After returning to civilian life with all its stresses and built-in sedentary habits, plus those home cooked meals, I started ballooning again into the high 190s.

I stopped myself before reaching 200, made a concerted effort based on the precepts of the BDS, and soon—and pretty permanently—was down to 175. Since that time, over ten years ago, I have stayed in the range of 175 to 185 pounds and still manage to eat the foods I like and enjoy.

I'm able to enjoy *life* much more, too. The BDS has enabled me to stop worrying about whether a diet is working, or whether it will get boring. I'm much more relaxed since I went on it, the kind of relaxation that refreshes you and gives you more energy for the things you want to do most.

Sensible diet-switching changed more than my weight. It changed my life. For the better. I think it will do the same for you.

3

Why Are We Overweight?

MOST DIETS EITHER TRY TO PSYCHOANALYZE YOU OR dismiss the question of why you're overweight completely, saying that if you do this and that, you no longer will be.

But why *are* you overweight?

I don't like that question. Because what it has come to mean basically is this: If you can find out the psychological reason for your extra pounds, then one-two-three, you won't overeat any more. Well, it's just not true, at least for over 90 percent of us. I've dealt with people who are overweight for a number of different reasons, so I would never say that there aren't psychological reasons for why we eat too much. There's a psychological reason for almost everything. But I've seen people go through ten years of intensive psychotherapy because they were obese, and come out obese.

One of the assets of the BDS—with the unusual exception of grossly overweight people, who indeed have either a real organic problem or a gross psychological disturbance—is that it doesn't matter why you're overweight.

(Severe psychological or organic disturbances as a cause of overweight are rare, and represent hardly more than 1 percent of the population. In these cases, dieting doesn't help, and more radical approaches must be taken. Intestinal bypass surgery is an example. But, again, this is so exceptional as to be virtually meaningless for you who are reading this book.)

Overeating can take so many forms, from the after-dinner snacker to the sweets lover to the meat-and-potatoes man, who many nights adds half a pound at dinner alone. And what they all have in common is this: Food tastes good. It's wonderful! It's probably the only accessible pleasure in life you can enjoy three times a day—every day.

That is why more than 90 percent of us overeat.

Yet the predominant school of psychological thought regarding overweight is best expressed by the "Don't-Be-Afraid-To-Be-Thin Diet." The idea is that we eat too much because we don't have a high enough opinion of ourselves. In other words, overweight is a form of self-deprecation.

Actually, I've found the opposite to be true most of the time. Food is a reward we give ourselves. You have to do something good—or be something good—in order to earn a reward, especially the reward of pleasure. Imagine a person—and there is a handful of these—who for physiological reasons cannot taste or smell food. How dreary would be much of this person's life compared to that of the rest of us!

Think if you couldn't even feel the sensation of hunger. You would probably perish. Thank goodness we have a tendency to overeat!

We Americans in particular have been made to feel guilty about the pleasure of eating. The majority of us think about and talk about food even more than we do about money and sex. Yet if you make a lot of money, do you feel guilty? If you make love most nights in the week, are you ashamed? On the contrary, that's a reason for bragging. But if you're 20 pounds overweight because you like food "too much," our society tries to make you feel you've done something terrible. Well, you haven't.

From a strictly medical standpoint, I can tell you with assurance that one of the first signs I look for in many an illness—and one of the first signs a psychiatrist looks for in chronic depression—is . . . loss of appetite. Columnist Mike Royko wrote not long ago about his visit to a German brat-wurst-and-beer emporium. He was struck by how much the people enjoyed themselves. Many were older folks and didn't look any the worse for it. Many also were a good 10 or 15 pounds overweight. Sure, it's true that you can try and eat your problems away and become overweight as a result of that. But there can also be a healthy overeating, and a healthy overweight. You're reading this book for two reasons—and the first is that you like food. All food! And that's a healthy thing.

The second reason is that you want to be slender. That's healthy too. But *only* if you keep your healthy appetite, and your love of the way the food you like tastes, because that is a crucial part of a love of the taste of life.

4

What Is Your Ideal Weight and Body Type?

BEFORE YOU START LOSING WEIGHT, YOU MUST KNOW how much weight you really should lose. Most people make the mistake of wanting to lose more weight than in fact they should.

One big reason for this is that we have a slimness mania in this country, which at times becomes actually a psychological illness, anorexia nervosa, when the individual literally almost starves to death because of a special preoccupation with being thin. Mainly overweight adolescents and mainly females, these individuals become unduly concerned about their weight and diet excessively to lose it. A phobia about food and a fear of a return to obesity leads to severe malnutrition and, in some instances, has even resulted,in starvation.

Few of us are really obese, which, medically, is said to be present when the body weight exceeds by 20 percent the standard weight listed in the usual height-weight tables.

Few of us go to the extreme of starvation. Still, few of us totally escape the obsession with slimness in America. A couple of years ago a musician in his fifties came to me because he had been about 30 pounds overweight for most of the last fifteen years. With the BDS he was able to lose those extra pounds within a matter of months, but he wouldn't stop there. "The Diet Switch isn't working any more," he told me.

"It's working," I told him. "You weigh about what you should. And the Diet Switch is keeping you there."

"No way," he said flippantly. "I want to lose 15 pounds more."

The only methods by which this man was realistically going to lose 15 pounds more were either to starve or to amputate a limb. For one thing, he was what is generally referred to as an endomorphic body type—and body types are the second big reason why most people miscalculate the amount of weight they should lose.

The identification some years ago of the three principal body types—ectomorph, mesomorph, and endomorph—was a step forward, I believe, which we haven't fully used. Not that any one person is all one type. But basically, the three are: a lean, high-strung ectomorph, protected against becoming overweight, at least until the middle years; the muscular, activity-minded, often larger-boned mesomorph; or the naturally heavier, more "rounded" endomorph, who will weigh 10 to 20 pounds more than another type of the same height no matter how hard he or she diets. One of the things that also seems true is that most people are *mixtures* of two types. In fact, I have seen a number of people who were basically of one type, but with this or that part of their anatomy a totally different body type. Many an ectomorph, for instance, has relatives who are endomorphs. In his twenties and even thirties he can eat twice as much as an ordinary endomorph or his mesomorphic neighbor and not gain an ounce. Then, in his forties, he will suddenly put on 10 or 15 pounds—but mostly in the abdominal area, possibly a few pounds around the face. His arms and legs will stay thin.

There is a definite physiological/anatomical basis for body types, however, and to know your ideal or truly normal weight, you have to get a handle on which one or combination you are. Ectomorphs are naturally thin, as I said, though some have a tendency to gain weight in one or two spots as the years pass. They are generally more high-strung, often "hyper," and this may be part of what makes them ectomorphs. Possibly their thyroid gland is set a little higher so that their metabolic rate burns up the food at a faster rate. Mesomorphs have more of their body weight taken up by bones and muscles. An ectomorph can exercise five hours a day to one hour for a mesomorph, and the mesomorph will still be more muscular. Probably because of this, mesomorphs have a higher physical energy level and enjoy activities that use their muscles and anatomy. Their problem is that with the onset of middle years much of the muscle may turn to fat unless the mesomorph keeps up his exercise or keeps a vigilant diet. The endomorph is a person with more fatty tissue, and actually has more cells per square inch in his body than a comparable mesomorph or ectomorph. The truly obese person does not have *more* cells in his body, but more *swollen* cells. The endomorph seems slightly more "swollen" than ectomorphs and mesomorphs because, even at his ideal weight, the endomorph has more cells and thus *should* weigh somewhat more.

Obesity is very seldom inherited. On the other hand, the heritability of somatotypes is strong. To be sure, obesity occurs more often in certain physical types, but in early life adipose tissue can grow by increasing both cell size *and* cell numbers. Once the number of adipocytes has been established, however, it does not seem to be susceptible to change. Therefore, in adult life obesity results solely from an increase in the size of the cells—which is what getting fat is all about. What this all adds up to, above and beyond body type itself, is the fact that you can lose weight more easily as an adult than as a child, because at least a number of your cells are not increasing, only the size of those cells.

There is another side to the coin of body types, though. It is that while some people are aware of their significance, many of us use them as excuses for overweight. An endomorph should weigh 10 to 15 pounds more than a similar mesomorph—but *only* 10 to 15 pounds more. A mesomorph who, because of a job or lifestyle, starts cutting down on the physical activities of younger years may say, "I can't understand why I'm gaining weight." And the ectomorph who used to be able to eat like a horse and whose tummy begins to resemble a cow at milking, suddenly looks down, sees the ballooning of that potbelly, and becomes angry that he can't eat quite like a horse any more without running like one.

It's pretty easy to tell which body type or types you are.

What you were like as a child is one indication. However, if you had an eating problem—if you were underfed or overfed—that may give a false picture. But simply a good look at yourself (you may have to take out an old photo) in a bathing suit or tennis shorts when you were last near your ideal weight gives a good indication. Mesomorphs, by the way, tend to have more pictures of themselves in bathing suits and tennis shorts. Their photos—as will a look in the mirror before getting dressed in the morning—reveal a more compact, rectangular build, with obvious physical strength. There seems to be a somewhat higher percentage of mesomorphic men than women, and a higher percentage of endomorphic women than men.

The endomorphic woman bears a similarity to the Titian woman. Even in childhood she had the cheek that the relatives always squeezed, and as an adult she may have the fanny that men like to pat. She has that extra bit of flesh here and there, and it's natural to her. The ectomorph, on the other hand, will always have parts of his or her body looking lean, even when overweight.

If you're still not sure what your basic body type is, ask yourself which relative you take after or "look like." And don't let the fact that Uncle Arthur was the black sheep of the family or that your mother was divorced three times stop you. We're talking only about anatomy, not morals or character.

A final insight about body types, nevertheless, is this: They aren't all there is to knowing your ideal weight. Dozens of factors enter into it—but don't worry about them. Except for those unusual people who have a metabolic problem (which your doctor would tell you upon a good, thorough checkup), those various factors don't add up to more than a few pounds one way or the other. If you're a couple of pounds underweight, fine. If you're a few pounds "over" weight, it's no big deal. The point is to be within a few. If your tummy is fairly flat, if you weigh within 10 pounds of what you weighed in your late teens or early twenties—and if you didn't have a weight problem then— that's good enough.

5

What Would You Like to Weigh?

IF YOU'LL TAKE A LOOK AT MOST POPULAR DIETS, you'll find that they really don't devote much thought to this question. Some of them merely give you a table in the back of the book, not unlike those old penny scales at Woolworth's that had a chart indicating average "normal" weights for men and women of so-called large, medium, and small body frames. They aren't that far off, mind you, but they aren't *that* exact either. Also, because they compute normal or desirable weights pretty much by fixed standards, their rather peremptory little listings lend an underlying, self-defeating, rotelike quality to their overall methods. It is as if they are saying, "Look, here's what you should weigh and everyone knows it."

24

What you feel from this, possibly unknowingly, is guilt. Because the inference is, "This is the way it is, the way it should be, and we all know it. Why haven't *you* done it?" Well, that *isn't* the way it is or should be. The Berkowitz Diet Switch is a way of guiding you permanently to the weight you want. Yet that doesn't necessarily mean that you have to be lean. If you're 15 pounds "overweight" and are satisfied, fine. Maybe you're 50 pounds overweight, which *is* too much, but want to lose only 30 of your 50. Again, fine. Dr. Robert Atkins rather grandiosely likened himself to Martin Luther King in saying, "Martin Luther King had a dream. I, too, have one." His "diet revolution" saw a world in which everyone was at his or her ideal weight. I don't have any such grandiose dreams, and I prefer evolutions to revolutions. I don't dream of a "world" in which everyone is this or that, because in my medical practice—and in my life—I have learned that each of us is an individual, and that the only "world" worth living in is one that permits each of us to follow and fulfill our own individuality.

Appendix A gives you a "range" of what you "should" weigh. This table—as all tables in this book unless I specifically indicate otherwise—is a collation of several of the most sensible guidelines in that area. The reason for this, especially when it comes to height and weight charts, is what I have been emphasizing: You can't pin it down within a pound or two. Even when we come to the calorie counts in foods, the best I can give you is a collation of the several most *nearly* correct statistics. How a specific food is cooked or packaged, where it comes from, and many other factors figure in. Consider the weight chart as a "ball park" figure. Use it as a midpoint, giving or taking a few pounds in either direction. Usually we know when we're about just the right weight because of how we feel—and because our tummy is fairly flat.

Two points: First, though there is a *range* of weights here, that doesn't mean that you should take the figures as a blank check. Let's say you're basically an ectomorphic type who'd like to think you're somewhat endomorphic. And let's say you're 5'6" tall. You might take the lower endomorphic figure of 127 pounds when you should really be taking the middle ectomorphic figure for that height and body build of 117.

That's a 10-pound difference. And 10 pounds you should not have.

But second, don't disregard other factors that may make a valid 3- or 4-pound difference. At different times of life— and I'm not talking about merely older and younger—we may put on or take off a few pounds almost "automatically." There is an inner metabolic reason for this, and it's something you shouldn't fight. It will adjust itself after a while. Of course, if you keep gaining or keep losing, you should sit up and take notice.

Illness can be another factor in weight gain or loss. Some people lose weight during a flu, while others eat too much and get out of bed 4 or 5 pounds heavier. Sometimes this is a good thing. You may need the extra food when you're ill. Again, you have to know yourself, and try and make it a matter of fitting your individual, healthy pattern, not merely indulge yourself.

Socioeconomic status and other economic factors influence the prevalence of overweight. In women especially, lower socioeconomic status shows overweight to be much more prevalent than in other groups. This is not to say that because you happen to be someone who doesn't make that much money right now, you have to weigh more than someone who does. Still, the structure of our lives does tend to influence us and cannot be disregarded completely.

So what would you like to weigh?

Don't base that figure on some article you read in a popular magazine, or what the neighbor down the street happens to look like, or some movie star. Base it on your own individualized situation and needs. The bottom line is your waistline.

If you can stand up straight, look down, and see all of your feet because your tummy is basically flat, you're very close to the right weight.

PART TWO

Diets
We Don't Use
and
Why

I know you're eager to get to the six diets that make up the Berkowitz Diet Switch. But before moving on to what the BDS is, it's important for you to know what it isn't.

That is because our human tendency is to want change for its own sake. Even some of my most successful patients who got down to their ideal weights on the BDS sometimes "added" an extra "diet." They figured if six were good, seven would be even better. The result was that they put a lot of weight right back on.

The six BDS diets, you see, are all balanced diets based on sound metabolic principles, each tailored to keep you happy with the food you eat while at the same time eating it in a way that will curb calories. I'm not saying that there doesn't exist another diet or two that could be added to our six, but in all the years I've been researching and testing the BDS I've never found it. I have found innumerable reducing plans that cannot sensibly be added to the BDS.

In the next dozen or so chapters we'll go briefly into just about every mode of diet that is either unhealthy, generally unworkable, or contains problems for those who want to lose weight permanently. This will enable you not only to understand better why the BDS works, but may tell you what you never knew about why diets you've tried before have invariably failed or failed to last.

31

6

Low Carbohydrate
Diets

THIS TYPE OF DIET HAS BECOME INCREASINGLY PREV-
alent in America in the last generation, and for a
good reason: We eat more carbohydrates than any people
in history. So, the reasoning goes, cut out a big chunk of
an American's carbohydrates, and you cut out a big chunk
of his overweight. A peak example of this is the Atkins Diet
of a few years ago, which advised us to eat virtually *no*
carbohydrates.

When taken out of context, as the Low Carbohydrates
(LC) diet often has been, the LC syllogism is unarguable:
(1) we're eating X number of carbohydrates; (2) X number
of carbohydrates is too much; therefore (3) eat less than X
carbohydrates and you'll lose weight.

But the context is crucial, and it reveals some overwhelming flaws. For one thing, most overweight individuals not only eat too much carbohydrate, they eat too much of *everything*. Eat too much of any type of food, even protein, and you'll be fat. Then what about the Atkins-type Diet, on which so many people temporarily lost weight? An almost no-carbohydrate diet works for awhile not because it's so good, but because the eating habits of a lot of people are bad. It's like the kid who is failing almost all his courses in school because he isn't paying attention in class or doing his homework. Have him pay attention for only a minute to get the assignment at the end of the class, and do just a quarter of an hour of homework at night, and he'll at least get Ds, maybe an occasional C. But he won't really be learning anything. School will be a less negative experience for him, yet still essentially negative. In the same way, cutting down on the excess amount of carbohydrates you are eating will make you lose weight no matter what else you eat or even how much of it for awhile. But in the long run you won't lose enough, and that loss is not all "healthy" pounds. Soon the average LC dieter is left with the prospect of cutting further not only on carbohydrates but on other foods as well.

The major problem with LC diets is that they put the cart before the horse—or the beef, if you will. They are disciplinary rather than supportive. And they are essentially negative, since their starting point is what you *don't* eat.

Moreover, they are telling you never ever to eat too many things you *like* to eat. On the BDS you may not be able to eat this or that for a few weeks, but we won't take a whole food group away from you. Even then, to the extent that we do take something away from you, it is always within the context of giving you something you *like*.

A final failing of the LC diets is that they are too limiting. Many foods and most menus are *mixtures* of protein, fat, and carbohydrates. So constructing a very low carbohydrate diet that can have a sustaining variety is very difficult. By eliminating too many foods with any appreciable amount of carbohydrates, you eliminate the joy of eating. Some of the BDS diets, it is true, give you fewer carbohydrates than you're used to, but you'll almost always have some of the ones you like. And the noncarbohydrate foods you'll eat are the ones you relish.

7

Natural Foods Diets

IN THE LAST DECADE THE NATURAL FOOD MOVEMENT HAS become a major nutritional phenomenon in our culture. All in all, a good thing it is, for the natural food philosophy has opened us up to the facts that (1) many of our foods contain substances which, taken even in minute quantities over a large quantity of years, can cause serious illness, and (2) many of our most popular foods do not contain significant nutritional values. But that doesn't mean that natural foods will help you lose weight.

Several neighbor couples, whom I first knew socially and who then used the BDS successfully, are an example. About seven years ago, when the "health food" craze was at its height, they began buying virtually everything from a natural food store. In three weeks the four couples gained an average of 11 pounds per person!

Realizing this, and still wanting to be as healthy as possible, they tried to find a way to put together natural foods with weight loss. They did not succeed. Today, about half their diet is natural foods, but half is not. However, they are at their ideal weight, which is worth its weight in naturalness.

Here's what happened: Three of the people, Marvin in particular, had a sweet tooth. This, they felt, was the essential reason for their being overweight. Walking into the health food store, they were confronted by those wonderful carob bars that contain no preservatives—but are certainly not short on calories! Being able to eat healthy "chocolate" for the first time was enough in itself to balloon them toward being overweight. However, there were other factors. Jan and Helen were snackers. Now they could snack on what was good for them physiologically—nuts, a variety of vitamin packed seeds, roasted soybeans, and the like. After a short time they were the most overweight of all. They had a variety of eating weaknesses, and it seemed that eating natural foods only accelerated those weaknesses. Why?

First, natural foods often contain more calories than their "unnatural" counterparts. Moreover, many of us eat "low cal" foods that indeed are heavy in preservatives and low in nutrition, and when we eat the same foods in their natural form, there are more calories within them because there is more nutrition in them. Second, since natural foods *are* natural, they stimulate our most fundamental physiological processes and actually increase our appetite. It's good to eat nourishing food, and our body responds by wanting more. Since we are not animals in a natural state, whose food must be struggled for physically in order to be eaten at all, the result is overweight.

So natural foods may tend to make you gain weight rather than lose it—if for some healthy reasons. What does that mean to you?

It means that although you may not be able to embark on a wholly natural diet and still trim your waistline, the more you use natural foods to replace the "same" artificial food, the better off you are. Few of the foods we eat these days are indeed "natural," yet most foods were once in a natural state. For instance, you'll never find a piece of white bread growing on a tree. For there to be a piece of white bread, at least a four-step process must take place to convert what grows in nature into bread. On the other hand, a head of lettuce will more or less go straight from the ground to you. A fish may go straight from the water to you.

Which brings us to the ultimate extension of the natural food movement—vegetarianism.

It is quite true that relatively few vegetarians are overweight. However, I look upon vegetarianism more as a philosophy than a weight-reducing regimen. If it happens to be your philosophy, you probably aren't reading this book. If you are a total vegetarian (no animal products of any kind) on ethical grounds, I consider that you may be giving up something at a sacrifice to you. What is given up when we eat no meat, fish, or dairy products at all is a combination of foods providing amino acids. Vegetarians are usually lean, but often wan. My experience has been that they do not as a rule have the same energy, and sometimes not the same all-round nutrition, as the typical American "meat-eater." On the other hand, the vegetarian is less subject to the health-damaging excesses of the typical American diet.

So, like low carbohydrate diets, "natural foods" and vegetarianism are used in the BDS not as diets, but as good ideas that should serve as an influence toward your selection of foods.

8

Willpower Diets

SOME TYPES OF DIETS ARE NOT VERY HELPFUL. ONE OF the diet types not useful for our purposes is what can be termed the "Straight Willpower" reducing methods.

Diminishing in popularity with every passing year—because if mere willpower worked, you wouldn't need a Willpower Diet—they still pop up in briefer forms in the pages of many leading magazines. Invariably, they contain two additional ingredients to make the medicine go down: (1) a basic, often healthy, lower calorie diet than you're used to, and (2) a minor twist, be it fruit for breakfast or vegetables for dinner.

Thus, the diet itself may *seem* a bit different, but this is only because the choice of foods in America is so huge that we'll never run out of variations on a fundamental formula. However, all of them boil down to a regimen of fewer calories than you're presently taking in. The key factor missing is that they don't really tell you how to stay on the diet. They only give you the diet and tell you that you'll lose weight with it. The invisible "how" is willpower—and it *is* invisible! Asking us to stay on a weight-reducing plan simply because we "should" is, in the long run, asking too much.

There's no point in discussing this type of diet in further detail. But it might be well to go to the heart of the matter and explain why willpower isn't practical. The big reason is that "willpower" isn't willpower. "Willpower" in diets is actually a red herring.

Our culture has come to place a tremendous premium upon free will, since we are the only creatures who have it in any significant way. I believe in free will. Not to believe that we have a choice is to disqualify ourselves from any growth or improvement. But the bottom line of free will is the *power* to *discover* and *adhere to* and *develop our true identities*. Two overwhelmingly important facets of your identity are (1) that you are not only a thinking being with free will, but an *animal* in the best sense of the word, who must conform to certain animal principles, and (2) your individuality as a total being.

The common fallacy about willpower—especially as it applies to dieting—is that it is the power to *do* something. Actually, willpower at its best means the power to *decide* something. In that sense, you have already decided something, and the most important "something" and the words you are reading now are the proof of it.

But you cannot "decide" to deny your animal nature, or your particular psychological needs and physiological tastes. In a word, the reason we're overweight, the reason we eat too much, the reason we have "bad" eating habits is because, first, we are animals who love and need food, and, second, we are *human* animals who love and need food!

The BDS wants you to keep being a healthy animal, and to stay as sweet as you are otherwise. Sure, you may have problems or weaknesses as we all do, but those are not the province of this book. As far as I'm concerned, all I know about you is that you're overweight and want to weigh less. Otherwise, you're perfect.

What I'm saying is that no, I don't want you to eat too much—most of the time anyway. I certainly don't want you to be overweight. And I don't want you to have bad eating habits that make you overweight. But we're going to accomplish these goals by *not* attempting to change your basic nature. Instead, the BDS will adapt that nature, will channel the things that make you eat too much or eat wrong so that you will lose those pounds. Willpower diets, in essence, try and change you, the *real* you.

Again, I know you're not perfect. Neither am I. But I don't know a single thing about you that is "bad"—except that you weigh too much. The Berkowitz Diet Switch can help you with that. And when you are down to your ideal weight, you won't have changed. You'll be more your real self. You'll again be what you were at your best. And, not surprisingly, you'll feel better equipped both physically and emotionally to deal with any other problems you have.

9

Fasting

ALMOST EVERYONE WHO HAS EVER BEEN MORE THAN a few pounds overweight, and wanted not to be, has sporadically fasted. Mention of this method goes back to the quasi-medical writings of ancient Rome and even to hieroglyphics. Sporadic Fasting can mean anything from a delayed breakfast to a deliberately missed dinner. Of all the popular diet types, it's the one that has been least publicized. The reason is that diet hucksters have found it unappealing. But limited fasting does have merit.

Misuse of the burgeoning study of nutrition has led us, falsely, to believe that physiologically we need "three squares a day." Well, it has been established that half a dozen small meals a day are superior to a couple of big ones—and, not incidentally, this is one of the six BDS diets.

On the other hand, missing a meal or skipping a snack can work—if you know how to do it. The Sporadic Faster who skips breakfast usually winds up with three cups of coffee and a doughnut (or similar intake) before lunch. Or, and this goes for light lunchers too, a mammoth dinner. And, often, a second dinner masquerading under the name of "snack" later on.

The tricks to what I call Sporadic Fasting are mostly common sense:

1. Know that that's what you're doing so that you don't eat a huge meal or snack later to cancel out the missed meal.

2. Realize that you're missing only a meal or two, and that you can eat a slightly larger meal afterward and still come out ahead. Whether we know it or not, down deep when most of us miss a meal, something inside whispers, "This is the way it's always going to be." And our instinct, both physiological and psychological, is to overeat to make up for it. If you firmly make a habit of thinking, "I'm going to miss only a single meal, two at the most," this will filter into your subconscious, and you won't have any trouble with Sporadic Fasting.

3. Pick the right time to miss a meal. If you're going to be doing some exercise, for example, it isn't likely that you'll be able to go for hours afterward without eating. On the other hand, let's say you know you're going to have dinner out one night. This may be a perfect opportunity to miss lunch. Then you can enjoy that big dinner, and if you be-

come a little hungry later on, eat a judicious but not fattening snack or two.

4. Drink a lot of water. This is not only for health reasons to avoid dehydration, but it fills you up and dilutes the stomach acids that catalyze hunger.

"Real," or extended, fasting is something else. Unless it's something you practiced successfully before, chances are you're neither physiologically nor psychologically fit for it. Most people, nutritional purists notwithstanding, should not fast for twenty-four hours or more. I know that some people swear by it, but in losing those two or three pounds when you go without eating for a day, you can also lose a little bit of your health. And, just as with Sporadic Fasting, you may tend to gorge yourself the following day. Even if you don't, extended fasting has this against it: It isn't a permanent way of losing weight. How long can you go without a meal?

Actually, fasting is a form of starvation. It goes against nature. Missing a meal or two to "clean the body out" does have merit. But even this may not be right for many of you. If you can do it successfully now and then, fine. If it's too difficult for you, that's fine too. Switching diets will accomplish what you want, without even a hint of starvation.

10

Dieting Through Hypnosis

ONE OF THE QUASI-MEDICAL DIET TYPES TO COME TO the forefront lately is hypnosis. Because hypnosis is founded on solid medical and psychological principles, it has been effective for a small but significant number of people. The principle is this: It conditions your subconscious mind against overeating. Even for those for whom it does not work permanently, it usually works for a time for everyone.

Above and beyond the fact that hypnosis, or subconscious suggestion, is now an accepted, valid medical/psychological tool, practiced by a number of doctors as well as therapists, it holds a second advantage that is different from most other diets: It assumes no willpower on your part.

Hypnosis is the only reasonable method that assumes even less willpower than the BDS. Yet this is also one of its drawbacks.

The prime problem with hypnosis is that it puts your overeating in the hands of somebody else. And maybe puts more than that in the hands of someone else.

Only future research will reveal all the reasons why hypnosis can be dangerous, but I think one—possibly the main one—is that tampering with the subconscious for a specific purpose while disregarding just about everything else is too tricky. The psychoanalyst deals with the subconscious, but hopefully in its entirety. The total person is brought forth. And the total *conscious* person is *there* to *see* and *hear* what's going on.

Hypnosis is also a mystery—to those who are hypnotized. As we've stressed more than once, the Diet Type which is unknown or unexplained to the dieter, is usually doomed to ultimate failure precisely for that reason.

There are other problems with hypnosis, but what they all add up to is this: Hypnosis is a specific quasi-medical/psychological treatment—which is somewhat analagous to surgical implantation—and it is a method that should be used *only* on those patients suited for it. I seriously doubt whether most of us are. Here I want to state outright my own prejudice against hypnosis: I myself don't like to be hypnotized, and never have been. I'm all for probing one's self-conscious, and tuning in on it to improve ourselves, but I don't like to lose control completely. Do you? In a minor way, hypnosis is like a general anesthetic, and this is something I would rather avoid if possible, both as a patient and a physician.

11

Aversion Diets

AVERSION METHODS OF DIETING ARE A KIND OF PHYS-
iological hypnosis, not unlike shock treatment. They
are against everything the Berkowitz Diet Switch stands for,
because their goal is to make you *dislike* what you *like!*

I can *see* using aversion methods for a problem like
smoking too much, because too many cigarettes are definitely a serious threat to health. And, of course, if one is
100 or 150 pounds overweight year after year, aversion
methods might be seriously considered, because people
who are consistently that obese may indeed have a psychological problem. This book is not for those who are
actually *obese*. It is for the vast majority of the American

public who are 15, 25, maybe 50 or somewhat more pounds overweight.

Of course, aversion methods can also work for a small percentage of people who are 30 to 50 pounds overweight. But on this subject I always think of Robert Ruark's epigraph to *Something of Value* that, "when you take away a man's customs, his traditions, his beliefs, you had better replace them with something of value."

It should be noted that there are some people in this world, though not many, who don't have a problem with overeating or overweight because they don't care that much about food. There are people, though not very many, who don't care that much about sex. I accept these people for what they are, but for the life of me I can't identify with them.

With the overwhelming majority of us, food is not only a value, it is a *necessary* value. The BDS is built upon the premise that you like food very much, or *love* it! Again, one of the differences between the BDS and other reducing plans is that here you don't have to feel the least guilt about loving food and loving to eat. You can be proud of it.

As we'll stress time and again, one part of life is inextricably bound to another: A good healthy appetite is mentally and physiologically part of being a good healthy person. Take away that appetite and the fulfillment of it, and you'll inevitably take away part of being a good healthy person.

This is why most people—yours truly included—have an aversion to aversion diets. So, in an effort to make this particular medicine go down, a half-brother of the aversion method has grown up in recent years: substitution methods. The idea here is to say, "Right, you should have an appetite for life and enjoy yourself. But not particularly where food is concerned—so try doing something else *more* and eating *less.*"

You may recall a substitution diet of a few years ago that was relatively short-lived. It advised substituting sexual activity for eating, the theory being that sex is an even more intense pleasure than food, so nothing would be lost in the substitution. It sounded good at first, to some people. At least in *theory.* One man who tried it told me, "I love sex, but this has turned my life upside down. I go to the office at seven-thirty in the morning and don't come home until six at night. They say you should run home for lunch and have a 'quickie' with your wife, but by the time I went there and back, it would take three hours, besides upsetting her day. And what was I supposed to do at the *end* of the day? Arrive home for a small meal and then jump into bed? I think the whole thing was a put-on, and I fell for it."

Physical exercise is another "substitution" that has been offered for eating. Get out on the handball court or jog or swim, we're told, and you won't want to eat as much. Nonsense. I'm all for physical activity because it is healthy for you. It puts more oxygen into your system, which not only uses up calories, but also seems to lead people toward eating more healthfully. Yet, whenever I get out on the tennis court for a couple of hours, I come away with a voracious appetite.

So what aversion and substitution methods add up to is a minus. They deny the fundamental thrust of our human psychology and physiology—to eat and to enjoy eating.

You can switch from one set of foods that you like to another. But you can't realistically switch from food to something else.

12

Diets That Support Your Weaknesses

ANOTHER TYPE OF DIET THAT COULD BECOME POPU-lar only in America is what I call the "Cater To Your One Weakness" reducing plan. I say only in America because, first, no country is as self-indulgent and permissive, particularly with food, as we are. And second, most countries do not have the affluence we have, permitting you to stuff yourself with your favorite delicacy in order to become thinner.

The epitome of this was the Caviar Diet of the late '60s.

Yet more realistic and better known is "The Drinking Man's" or "Busy Exec's" Diets. There is gold in this idea, but not in the diets themselves.

The valid idea behind these diets—for many people—is

that we who are overweight are only human and, especially when it comes to the enormous gratification that food gives, will always have some "weakness" that will result in excess pounds if we don't find a way to deal with it. The Drinking Man's Diet, for instance, addressed itself to the 35 million or so Americans for whom alcohol is a regular and calorically significant part of their menus. As a practicing physician, I will say something most doctors wouldn't: If you tell these 35 million men and women simply to cut down on (or cut out) their drinking, you'll have failed them, at least as far as being overweight is concerned. Moreover, you may be failing many of them as far as good health is concerned.

Sure, excessive alcoholic intake is not good for you. But most people who take in 1,500 calories weekly or more in alcohol (or drinks mixed with alcohol) have a good reason—for *them.* Yes, maybe they would live several years longer if they didn't drink as much; maybe they'd feel better if they didn't drink at all.

Maybe.

And maybe not.

Scientific studies are contradictory on this. Some studies show that those who imbibe 2 to 6 ounces of alcohol daily—though no more—live significantly longer than total abstainers. Why would this be?

There are several reasons. To begin with, we do know scientifically that small or moderate amounts of alcohol have beneficial effects on the heart, circulation, and digestion. Alcohol is one of the oldest "drugs" and can indeed be used for medicinal purposes. Second, there is little doubt that the proper use of alcohol can be tranquilizing. In the chaotic world into which we are thrust, a good tranquilizer shouldn't be undervalued. Third, moderate drinking may be part of a lifestyle which, all in all, is healthier for certain people than the alternate lifestyles open to them.

The prudent physician must look at the total human being. Not long ago I was invited for dinner at the home of a man who has been my patient for more than ten years. It was a family-type occasion, and he had both his married children and his own parents there. Before eating, both the grandmother and grandfather almost religiously drank two large glasses of wine. "We have only missed our wine before dinner three times in our marriage," the smiling gentleman said. He also revealed later that he began the day with a shot of schnapps. "It gets me going," he said. "My father did it before me." The man's father had lived to 86. He was 81, and his wife was in her late seventies. They appeared robust and in good health.

Closer to home for most of us is Edward R. Ed is a busy businessman in his early forties. The last thing he'd think of doing is have a "morning" drink, but the first thing he does upon coming home in the evening is to mix himself a high highball. He sips it while talking to his wife about the day, and it puts him in a better frame of mind for his kids and the dinner they all subsequently enjoy together. Several times a week he also has a couple of martinis at a business lunch. Under financial pressure, as are so many of us with the economy the way it is, would it be realistic to say that Ed should let up in his high-pressure job, simply take a deep breath before a business lunch, and then do some yoga when he walks into the house after a day of battling the world? No way. One of the most obvious alternatives for Ed and so many like him is to pop tranquilizers during the day, rush through lunch, and walk through the front door at night shouting "Don't anyone talk to me! I've had a terrible day!" And from there plunge into an argument with his wife and create problems with his children.

On the other hand, there are a lot of men and women who drink a lot more than Edward R. and the octogenarian couple. It isn't good for them. But no diet is going to solve their problem drinking or alcoholism for them. Edward and the older couple don't need a "drinking diet," because they've already sensibly built drinking *into* their diets. On the other hand, the problem drinker has built his diet around drinking. Moreover, he invariable has other problems besides alcohol.

So, "The Drinking Man's Diet," "The Busy Exec's Diet," and the other "Cater To Your One Weakness" reducing plans don't work because they take a premise that is true and apply it in a way that is untrue for the vast majority of us. They also make a fatal assumption—that we have only *one* weakness.

As I mentioned earlier, I'm of a body type prone to be 8 to 10 pounds overweight, but no more. But those 8 to 10 pounds were a recurring problem for me until I went on my own Diet Switch. Though most people who are overweight are in the 16 to 25 or 26 to 49-pound range, that makes me even a better example of why working with only one weakness won't work. I, for instance, have *three* weaknesses when it comes to food.

Another problem with the "Cater To Your One Weakness" diets is that the reducing plan itself is seldom much of anything. What they really do is give you some of your "poison," then build a reduced calorie, balanced diet around that. And the same ultimate failure will come about from this diet as from any other. Moreover, as we've emphasized, your "poison" often isn't poison at all. And when it is, because it plays too important a part in your caloric intake, you need more than a diet to deal with it.

The Berkowitz Diet Switch may help you get a handle on other problems in your life. But the only problem it solves directly is the problem of overweight.

13

"Somehow" Diets

ONE OF THE MOST PREDOMINANT TYPES OF DIETS IN recent years has been the Somehow Diet. No one knows precisely why it works, but it does work somehow, we're told, and that's all we should care about.

Well, assuming that a Somehow Diet isn't dangerous, it *doesn't* work permanently for most people. And it *is* important to know why it works.

These diets often do work for many people for awhile, but for the reason we talked about at the outset: *Any* diet will work for awhile simply because you're on a diet.

However, for the vast majority of us, they succeed less and less with each passing week after the initial honeymoon. And the crucial reason this type of diet doesn't work is precisely because you do not know what makes it "work."

For awhile there's an alluring mystery to that. There's something in each of us that yearns for a true miracle. The Berkowitz Diet Switch is no miracle, and is called that only within the context of all the diets that haven't worked for you. However, I know why BDS works, and if you don't know why a Somehow Diet is supposed to succeed, slowly but inexorably your confidence in it will be eroded, and a mistrust will replace the mystery.

So, when it comes to a permanent way of eating which will make you lose that excess weight and keep it off, we'll save our mysteries for reading Agatha Christie. There is ultimately *nothing* to recommend a Somehow Diet as a permanent reducing method. Thus it is not one of the types which you'll be using on the Switch.

Enough of Somehow.

How is better.

14

Liquid Diets

L IQUID DIETS ARE NOT INCLUDED IN THE BDS, MAINLY because few people can tolerate them. Oh, I'm sure that somebody's sister-in-law has told you grand stories of how she lost 15 pounds in a week or two on some commercial liquid diet. And no doubt she did. It's even possible to put together a liquid diet that you don't have to buy in a store that will fill your nutritive needs and make you lose weight. But I've found the percentage of people who could stick to something like this even for a week or two so low that it wasn't realistic to include a liquid diet in our plan.

Also, there are a couple of rather large minuses against liquid diets. One is that they aren't healthy for your intestinal system, even over short periods of time. More and more, we're finding out that a certain amount of roughage is needed to clean out the colon in particular. Studies have shown that cruciferous vegetables in the diet—such as brussels sprouts, cabbage, broccoli and others—may actually be a preventive against colon cancer, which is one of our greatest killers. These vegetables seem to clean out the colon by possibly preventing the formation of polyps which can later turn malignant. But above and beyond that, liquid diets are simply not a natural way of eating for adults, because a liquid diet isn't eating, it's drinking.

Also a dependence upon liquid diets seems to develop in many people who have tried them. Several factors account for this. Most liquid diets are sweet, and thus mildy addictive to those with a sweet tooth. They are easily accessible, and require little preparation. They allow you to satisfy your hunger throughout the day and evening—a little liquid here and a little there (and maybe *more* than a little here and there). Whatever the reason, a significant percentage of people who try liquid diets continue past the point where they need to, it's better not to get into the habit.

Before leaving liquid diets, though, it's important to say something about liquids *in* your diet—any diet. The right liquids do tend to help us in almost all diets, and promote weight loss. That was the genius of Dr. Stillman's "water diet." The menus in his reducing regimens were not extraordinary. But by insisting that the individual drink a goodly number of glasses of water each day, the Stillman Diet gained at least temporarily good results that most diets don't. Water has no calories, tends to fill us up, and also dilutes the stomach acid that helps to make us hungry. There's evidence, too, that water with most meals—as long as you don't overdo it—may have a catalytic effect, especially when protein and fat are eaten together with carbohydrates, that helps burn up calories.

However, there are liquids and there are *liquids*. So, though I do advise you to drink liberally on virtually all of the BDS diets, this does not mean that you can go heavy on any type of liquid other than water. Here's a thumbnail assessment of the major beverages:

—*Milk.* American adults who are "milk drinkers" seldom need as much as they consume. Doctors have even begun to see that children in this country may be drinking far more milk than is good for them. Milk has calories, milk has cholesterol, and milk is very allergy-producing in many people. Because they don't break out in hives or sneeze, people may not realize that their indigestion is due to their milk drinking. In any event, *though milk can be a part of a number of BDS diets, it is NOT a liquid to fill up on between meals.*

—*Malted milks and shakes.* These are a one-way ticket to obesity. On a couple of our diets you may indeed drink malted milks, but they are a far cry from a glass of water and *must* be *part* of a meal, not considered a liquid per se.

—*High protein drinks.* I'll never forget when a friend of mine went on a high protein "health food" diet. At the center of it was a high protein drink he consumed half a dozen times daily. It consisted of skim milk (which, though lower in calories than ordinary milk, has a high percentage of carbohydrates that offsets the whole high-protein principle), a couple of heaping teaspoons of the protein mix, and a few teaspoons of sugar to make the drink palatable, even lovable. Six feet tall with an average frame, George weighed 182 when he began this high protein diet. A month later he weighed 206. He couldn't understand it. But I could. He had taken out of context the fact that a high protein diet theoretically burns up fat and reduces your weight. He wasn't cutting down that much on his meals; he was simply adding the protein drink to them. And those protein drinks contain quite a few calories, with the milk and sugar, to say nothing of the heaping teaspoons of protein itself! Moreover, six glasses a day was like six small meals a day, in addition to whatever else he was eating.

To sum up, I think an occasional drink of a high protein mix—even one or two a day, depending upon the diet you're on—can be good for you. But again, it must be part of your daily menu. It isn't some magical, liquid extra that will temporarily fill you up without putting on calories.

—*Colas. Playboy* publisher Hugh Hefner has been known to drink fifteen cola drinks a day most days of the week and stay rail thin. In all likelihood this is because he has that unusual kind of metabolism that burns up calories. Just looking at him the first time I was at the Playboy mansion, I noted that Heff appeared to be near the classic ectomorphic body-type that almost never gets fat. This isn't true of most of the rest of us. If you drink only an occasional cola now and then, you can consider it a liquid that, though containing some calories, isn't a part of your diet. But most cola drinkers seem to drink three or four a day, and this definitely falls into the category of a food that will add weight.

—*Diet colas.* Though the saccharin and cyclamate et al. controversy still rages and is unresolved, and though these drinks do not put on weight, I'm against overusing them as a way of keeping weight down. I believe in playing it safe, and the safety of too many of these diet drinks (in terms of whether they cause dangerous chemical changes in the body) is still a real probability. Again, one every day or two shouldn't hurt you. But drinking them on a regular basis could add up to a great hazard over the course of years.

—*Coffee.* A very small percentage of people who drink coffee take only a cup or two a day. If you do, even with cream and sugar, this shouldn't figure prominently in up-setting any of your BDS diets. But if two becomes three or four or more, and you take cream and sugar, you will put on some extra weight. Not to mention the fact that too much coffee can have other ill effects on your health.

—*Tea.* It's difficult to categorize tea. There are some people who load it with sugar and cream and drink a dozen cups a day and wonder why they can't get their weight down. Generally, though, if you're not this kind of tea drinker, this can be an ideal between-meal liquid, either iced or hot.

—*Hard liquor.* As we said at the outset, the Berkowitz Diet Switch isn't designed to *change* you; it's a food-wise diet designed to take you as you are and show you a better way of dealing with problem weight. If you like your hard liquor, for example, none of the diets you'll be on will ask you to give it up. There are many people who are not problem drinkers or alcoholics (and problem drinkers and alcoholics almost always can use a better diet) who have occasional drinks at lunch and/or before dinner, possibly a highball before they go to bed. Or they drink little throughout the week but heavily on the weekend when they socialize. This can be lived with. But what you do have to know from a reducing standpoint is how many calories you're drinking. Half a dozen "grasshoppers" a week will make your scale jump. Consult tables in Appendix B on the caloric count of different drinks, and generally use this rule of thumb: If the hard liquor you're drinking adds up to more than 200 calories a week, consider it as part of your diet. If not, enjoy.

—*Beer*. Beer is a food. As a matter of fact, it isn't a bad food, in moderation. But it *is* a *food*.

—*Fruit juices*. Here you can gauge whether these can be considered a food or a liquid, pretty much the way you gauged hard liquor intake. Some fruit juices have a lot more calories than others. They are healthier for you than liquor, though. So if you can use them in moderation and stay below 200 calories a week, fine.

—*Flavored drinks*. By these I mean the commercial products where you mix a teaspoon or two with water (and sometimes more than a little sugar). Some of them advertise that they contain huge amounts of Vitamin C and so forth. Indeed they do, or they couldn't advertise it, but don't forget that vitamins are derived from different sources and that the best, most effective way to vitaminize your system is by getting those vitamins and minerals through the foods you eat, or a top-grade multivitamin pill. Flavored drinks *can* generally be considered liquids and not part of your food intake. But be careful to read the labels. They may contain a lot more than the flavor—not in calories necessarily, but in chemical additives. And take note of how much sugar you put in.

—*Cocoa-flavored drinks*. These almost always contain

enough calories to be considered a food. Moreover, because they are so sweet and temporarily filling, cocoa-type drinks—while they can be a wonderful *part* of most diets—tend to upset the diet you are on if taken haphazardly. It's not that you have to worry about one or two of this or that during the course of a week. But most people tend to favor two or three kinds of beverages. If this is one of those you like, let's build it into your diet instead of your waistline measurement.

—*Concoctions and other "liquids."* We can't go into all the minor drinks, nor do we need to. If you are regularly taking in some other liquid other than the above, figure out how many calories go into it and act accordingly. I might say something about "concoctions" that people make for themselves.

"Concoctions" are merely individualized beverages that people concoct for themselves. The reason may be health, as in herbal drinks, or it could be weight loss. In either case you must beware of how many calories are going into the concoction. Also, don't accept "Grandma's old elixir" just because Grandma was never overweight or lived to be 90. A lot of concoctions are handed down, and it would be better if they were thrown out.

15

Etceteras

THERE ARE MANY SPECIFIC DIETS THAT WE HAVEN'T covered here. But there are no significant omissions, because any we have not touched on are related pretty closely to at least one that we have. The only exception might be the group dieting method, which has become quite popular in recent years.

Although I would not dispute that a great many people lose a great deal of weight on group diets, as a physician I hold the puristic feeling that the group is more of a crutch, like hypnosis or diet pills, than a permanent way to lose weight. Must you go to the group forever? I don't think this is good or realistic.

There are a number of people, it is true, who have lost weight merely by following the diet given by this group or that, without ever attending the group itself. This simply supports our thesis that any good diet, followed diligently, will make you lose weight. But will it do so over the years ahead?

As with a number of other diet types that have worked and that can be adapted to your purpose, there is good sense in the "group diet" you can apply *without* going to a group. It is this: What others think of us can be a motivation. It's good to have one or more people around who say, "Hey, you lost some weight" or "You look real good—have you lost weight?" You will hear such comments once you're on the BDS for a short time. But if you know someone else or a number of people who are on the BDS, it does help to *see* them and give that support to one another. Some people who have gone on the Berkowitz Diet Switch have persuaded others to try it, and their "group" success does tend to give them a little extra boost.

In the final analysis, however, you are alone with your own mirror, you own scale. Your own motivation must suffice—and it will.

Enough said about other diets. Let's move on to the BDS diets, about which by now you are probably curious, to say the least.

PART THREE

The Berkowitz Diet Switch Diets

16

The High Protein
Diet

T HE FIRST OF THE SIX BDS DIETS IS THE HIGH PROTEIN
diet. Three excellent assets of this diet are: (1) It's
basically very healthy for you; (2) it gives more immediate
weight loss than most of the other diets; and (3) chances
are you'll love it.

Protein is basically healthy for us because it provides the
building block of our physiology. Also it filters through the
body at a steady rate over a number of hours, so the feeling
of needing food doesn't burgeon again until it's time for the
next meal.

The High Protein Diet gives more immediate weight loss
than most of the other BDS diets because, to put it sim-

plistically, it is the nature of protein to be used for the bodily tissues themselves rather than to be stored. A high protein diet, especially when it is low in carbohydrates, tends to "burn itself up" more. Also, the overwhelming percentage of people who are overweight have eaten too many carbohydrates or fats. A high protein diet is, therefore, generally the best to start out with because the reduction of fats and carbohydrates, when replaced by protein, often gives a dramatic weight loss and starts off the journey toward normal weight on an encouraging note.

Finally, the chances are that you'll love the High Protein Diet, since most of us in America are protein-eaters from an early age. This goes far past loving a good steak or a hamburger. When you stop to think about it, so many foods Americans like begin with protein. The trouble is that too much carbohydrate is added to it. Like the sausage pizza. Some people simply will not eat a plain cheese pizza, but will eat a sausage pizza. Unfortunately, they are getting many times more carbohydrates than the protein of the sausage. The same goes for a hot dog, where the bun has more calories than what's inside it. Spaghetti and meatballs is another example. What I try to do with my own kids is to accustom them to eating the hamburger without the roll, and the same with the hot dog. They can have all the trimmings they want, except for the bread. Actually, onions and relish and tomatoes are fine for you. When you eat at an Italian restaurant, better to have extra meatballs and go slow on the spaghetti or, even better, forget it.

One of the good things that will happen to you through the BDS is that you'll get used to eating better foods. You'll still have your hamburger, but oftener than not you won't have the hamburger roll. Which is fine, if you really like hamburger. If you don't, why not get rid of the hamburger habit altogether and eat something you do like that isn't fattening.

At the end of this chapter I'm going to give you a list of the most common high protein foods. I'm not going to waste pages and insult your intelligence by going into an assiduous list of every possible protein food, from stewed Abyssinian albacore (if there is such a thing) to Tibetan trilobite (if there ever was such a thing). For fifty cents you can buy one of those little pamphlets that tell you the calorie counts of every possible food ever conceived. If you've been overweight for any reasonable amount of time, you probably have one.

Nor am I going to give you menus. I'm not going to tell you what you like to eat.

But while on the High Protein Diet at least two-thirds of the calories you consume should be protein.

Other than that, the more balanced and healthy the carbohydrates and fats you eat, the better off you'll be. And you know very well what's healthy. Bear in mind that you're free to choose what you want for the calories other than protein. But don't push the protein much farther than two-thirds. You do need some carbohydrates and fats also.

A word of advice here: The High Protein Diet works best when that nearly 70 percent of your calories in protein is eaten every day rather than averaged out over two or three days. For instance, if you eat only 40 percent protein on Monday and try and make up for it with 95 percent on Tuesday, your weight loss will be less than if you were at 65 percent or 70 percent of calories in protein each day.

Two weeks is the usual time for staying on the High Protein Diet before switching to the next in order. Since it offers considerable variety, most people do not tire of it easily.

Most Common High Protein Foods

	Calories
Dairy Foods	
American cheese (1 oz.)	106
Cottage cheese, creamed (1 oz.)	35
Eggs (1, soft-boiled or poached)	80
Fish and Seafood	
Clams (canned, 4 oz.)	90
Crabmeat (1 cup)	102
Flounder (4 oz.)	80
Ocean perch (fried, 4 oz.)	255
Sardines (canned, 4 oz.)	350
Shrimp, fresh (fried, 4 oz.)	250
Tuna (canned, 3 oz.)	325
Fowl	
Chicken breast (1 average, broiled)	152
Turkey, light meat (roasted, 4 oz.)	210
Meat	
Bacon (2 slices)	88
Beef roast (1 slice, about 5 oz.)	202
Beefsteak (broiled, 5 oz.)	575
Ham (3 oz.)	340
Hamburger (broiled, 4 oz.)	245
Lamb chop (1, broiled)	375

	Calories
Liver, beef (fried, 3 oz.)	200
Pork chop (broiled, 1 thick)	440
Veal cutlet (broiled, 1)	155

Nuts

Almonds (1 cup)	850
Cashew nuts (1 oz.)	165
Peanut butter (1 tbsp.)	95

Sausage

Bologna (4 oz.)	320
Frankfurter (1)	130
Pork links (3)	210

Vegetables

Beans, green (1 cup)	32
Beans, with pork and tomato sauce (1 cup)	304

Super High Protein Mix

(With one 8 oz., 164-calorie glass of whole milk)	274

17

The Bare Breakfast, Little Lunch, and Deal-With-Dinner Diet

REDUCING PLANS ALMOST INVARIABLY HAVE BEEN LIKE the two sides of the Grand Canyon. One side tells you to eat certain foods, day in and day out, year in and year out, and you'll lose weight. The other side tells you to eat less, and you'll lose weight. Both sides are "correct." But the huge hole in the middle for both is that they don't tell you *how*.

My experience—and no doubt yours—shows that the first is an impossibility. If you could eat an essentially healthy diet of certain foods that would reduce you down to your ideal weight, year after year, you would have been doing it in the first place and wouldn't need that particular reducing plan! As we've pointed out consistently, people seldom want to eat the same group of foods year in and year out. It takes the enjoyment out of eating, becomes boring, and eventually even hateful. It simply isn't workable for close to 99 percent of those who are overweight.

The obvious alternative, according to most "experts," is to eat a variety of foods, but not as much of them. Again, you knew this was an answer since the first time your waistline began to expand. You tried it, and eventually it didn't work either. You once more fell into the Grand Canyon of overweight, because the question of *how* effectively to eat less was never really answered.

The Bare Breakfast, Little Lunch, And Deal-With-Dinner Diet supplies an answer.

The crucial *how* of the Bare Breakfast, Little Lunch, and Deal-With-Dinner Diet is that you don't have to follow it forever. Two weeks, even one—in some cases, even a couple of days—is all that you need. Knowing that months or a lifetime of eating less *isn't* staring you in the stomach, you can do this for a couple of weeks, certainly a couple of days.

First, let's zero in on why the Bare Breakfast, Little Lunch, and Deal-With-Dinner Diet works so well for most people, by talking briefly about those for whom it *doesn't* work well.

What about a healthy breakfast being the most important meal of the day? Well, though there's definitely something to this metabolically, our two hundred-year-old belief in a hearty breakfast stems from a time when most men and their wives farmed or labored physically much of the day, and overweight was the exception rather than the rule. Today, the situation is reversed. Most men and women go off to desk jobs, are in their cars much of the day, with push-button devices surrounding them, so that even when they have to "do" something, it doesn't take a tenth of the physical effort it once did. Even many "physical" jobs have been made partly sedentary or automated, and the average person in such trades is likely as not to be overweight. What it adds up to is this: Few of us need a big breakfast any more. We should have some breakfast, but the kind of hearty opening meal of the day that has long been accepted as good for you can actually make you feel bloated, even somewhat fatigued. And it unquestionably contributes to being overweight.

The Bare Breakfast part of this diet should consist of two things:

1. No more than 15 percent of your daily caloric intake, possibly as low as 10 percent.
2. Whatever you enjoy eating, but preferably just one food, possibly with a beverage.

But is that a balanced breakfast? Of course it isn't. One of the most common mistakes we make is to think we have to balance each meal. We don't. We have only to get a basically balanced diet from the whole day, or even out of every two days.

Here are some sample breakfasts that have been used on this BDS diet:

—A couple of strips of bacon and juice
—Several eggs (with the yellow removed), topped with a little salad dressing
—A couple of teaspoons of peanut butter sprinkled lightly with honey

—A piece of toast, not heavily buttered
—Fresh or canned fruit and Rye Krisp
—A small salad
—You get the idea.

The point is that you can eat *anything* for breakfast, as long as it doesn't exceed your percentage of calories. It's better to eat a breakfast of cooked egg whites, because, as eggs are high in protein, they will continue to filter throughout your body throughout the morning, and you won't get hunger pains an hour or two later, as often happens with a high carbohydrate breakfast. If you do choose a breakfast mainly of carbohydrates, prepare yourself for a midmorning snack, and make sure it merely fills you up, not fills you out.

The Bare Breakfast, Little Lunch, and Deal-With-Dinner Diet, you see, is good for both the person who skips breakfast and the person who goes too heavy on breakfast. The breakfast-skipper may think he or she is saving calories, but will almost always make it up by midmorning or at lunch— at dinner for sure. Better to eat a small breakfast that makes that sometimes high-calorie midmorning snack or large lunch unnecessary.

The big breakfast eater—unless he's that unusual individual who is able to have his biggest meal of the day in the morning—gets off to a bad start. A social lunch, not pushing away from the table at dinner, a midnight snack— and a pound or two for the day has been added. Maybe some days it doesn't happen. But some days it does. With a small breakfast, you know you have that "reserve" of calories in case lunch or dinner gets out of hand.

So let's say you've eaten that small breakfast, possibly

added 50 or 100 calories at midmorning, and now are confronted with lunch. Here are the guidelines for lunch:

1. It should contain no more than 20 percent of your total calories for the day.
2. Try and schedule your lunch later than usual, but not so late that you're *extremely* hungry.

For most of us it isn't necessary—either for nutrition or for gratification—to eat that large a lunch. We do it out of habit, because of a social situation, or for some other unsubstantial reason. If you have a little breakfast, and you have dinner to look forward to, you can handle lunch if only you're aware that this is where too many calories are accumulating.

And . . . if you've eaten a minimal breakfast and a small lunch, you *can* deal with dinner. How?

First of all, many of you won't have to deal with it—you'll just be able to enjoy it!

There are two kinds of dinner eaters. Some of us are among the many that like a good, full evening meal, and are satisfied once we've had it (notwithstanding a minor snack or two later). Well, if this is you, it will be a real boon to find that you have 65 percent to 70 percent of your caloric intake for that day left for the evening meal!

Don't use it all up, though. Allow 5 percent, or 6 percent, or 8 percent for that snack later on.

The other kind of dinner eater is the Buddy Hackett type. The famous comedian once said how he could pass up breakfast and lunch rather easily, "and then eat half of Omaha for dinner."

A lot of people fall into this category, but here are some guidelines for dealing with dinner:

1. Eat slowly. I realize this is easier said than done, unless you know how. By eating slowly, I don't mean to chew your food slowly, reach for a second helping slowly, and that nonsense. If you have to think *how* you eat *while* you're eating, it takes all the enjoyment out of it. And if you can't enjoy dinner, what can you enjoy in life? Instead, though, if you're eating with your family, set more time aside for dinner. Make conversation a part of your meal. Try and have a leisurely meal out with friends or on the patio or porch whenever you can. And if you're alone, bring a book to the table or tune on the TV and take your time.

2. Schedule dinner a little later. You're going to be hungry anyway, so you might as well eliminate that *big* snack later by getting filled up at seven or seven-thirty rather than five-thirty or six.

3. Average out your calorie count for dinner over two or even three days. In other words, don't be afraid to eat a really big dinner every couple of days or so. Just go a little lighter the next day, while still eating a full nighttime meal.

The Bare Breakfast, Little Lunch, and Deal-With-Dinner Diet, you'll find, begins to work quite well after the first few days. In the very beginning, don't expect dramatic results. What you're actually doing here is modifying your behavior somewhat, changing your habits somewhat, and it takes some time to get into that. Once you do, though, you'll find that it *is* becoming a habit and that your second week will show a good deal of weight loss. This may be one of the diets, in fact, that you'll want to continue for longer than two weeks.

18

The Fill-Up-On-Salad-Or-Something-Similar Diet

N O DIET IS NEW. AND ONE OF THE OLDEST KINDS IS THE Fill-Up-On-Salad-Or-Something-Similar Diet. This method for dealing with overweight goes back to some of the earliest recorded civilizations. Yet every year or two somebody comes up with a slight variation on it, and it's labeled the "breakthrough" or "most original" reducing plan of the century.

Actually, the Fill-Up-On-Salad-Or-Something-Similar Diet is only common sense. It's like this: You're overweight. The reason you're overweight is that you eat too much of some foods that have too many calories. That leaves you only two choices as far as eating is concerned: (1) eat less, or

(2) eat food that has less calories. It's hard to eat less, so what's left is to eat foods that have less calories more often.

Of course, if it were *that* simple, this would be the only diet anyone would ever need. It isn't that simple, and that's precisely why we have the BDS. What switching accomplishes is, first and foremost, to allay boredom and supplant "willpower." And there is seldom anything more boring than eating a lot of salad or something similar day after day, year after year. Even eating your favorite foods day in and day out gets to be a bore and a chore—and salad-type foods are seldom our favorite food. On the other hand, you may find that the Fill-Up-On-Salad-Or-Something-Similar diet gives you a taste for salads you haven't had before. Many BDSers, after completing their switch to the Fill-Up-On-Salad, etc., Diet, came away with a real liking for low calorie foods that filled them up. They were then able more easily to make salads, and so forth, a part of the next (or some subsequent) diet to which they switched.

There are all kinds of salads. You can't drop a steak onto the lettuce, but chances are overwhelming that one dressing or another will be to your liking because many dressings are based upon foods that you probably like—such as cheese. There is no law against using more than one dressing on a salad, either. Or putting little cut-up bits of your favorite food in there—and it could be cold steak. The point is to make these salads you eat between meals and for some of your meals as interesting and tasty to you as possible, while keeping the calories down. You fill up, but you don't fill out.

Some of you, however, will say, "I simply hate salads." What you probably hate is lettuce. Well, lettuce doesn't have to be the basis of a salad. Use celery. Or anything that is low in calories and can serve as a condiment for the dressing you're putting on it or whatever other food you're sprinkling in it.

Following is a brief list of the foods most naturally adapted to the BDS Diet No. 3:

Most Common Fill-Yourself-Up Foods

	Calories
Carrots, raw (1 average)	20
Celery, raw (1 average stalk)	8
Collards (boiled, ½ cup)	31
Cucumbers:	
With skin (1 average)	35
Peeled (1 average)	29
Kumquats (1 average)	11
Lettuce:	
Boston or Bibb (½ head)	11
Iceberg (½ head)	36
Romaine (6 leaves)	11
Onions, raw (1 average)	38
Parsley, raw (½ cup)	11
Pepper, sweet green, raw (1 average)	15
Pickles:	
Dill (1 large)	14
Bread and butter (4 slices)	20
Sour (1 large)	13
Sweet gherkin (1 small)	20

	Calories
Radishes, raw (5 medium)	4
Spinach (boiled, ½ cup)	20
Tomatoes, raw (1 medium)	18
Zucchini (boiled, ½ cup)	10
Water	0

You'll notice that water is included on the list. I realize that it's no great culinary treat to drink water. But a few glasses between meals—or low-cal beverages (as I mentioned, I don't like low-cal beverages consistently, but for a couple of weeks, no problem) can also fill you up temporarily so that you'll avoid high calorie snacking. When you do snack on food, however, try and make it a few celery sticks with salad dressing or maybe a little peanut butter, that kind of thing.

The Fill-Up-On-Salad-Or-Something-Similar Diet doesn't mean that you won't eat other foods besides the salads or things from a similar group. But the guideline here is that at least half your calories should be the low-cal foods that fit this diet. You'll find that that's an awful lot of food, and that you'll feel quite full virtually all of the time. You'll get enough of what you like with the remaining calories so that you don't feel at all starved or bored. However, a couple of weeks of this—less in many cases—is the most that the majority of us can take. That's why it's often good to follow up this diet with one of the others you like very much, such as the Sweet-Tooth Diet.

19

The Sweet-Tooth Diet

"I WISH I COULD JUST EAT SWEETS FOR A WEEK AND satisfy my sweet tooth once and for all."

I've heard this, give or take a word or two, from the majority of men and women whose main reason for overweight is that they eat too many sweets. Years ago, comedian Jackie Gleason was known for saying with the greatest of gusto, "Oh, how *sweee—eee—eet* it is!" The meaning of that phrase, of course, is how *good* it is. He used the word "sweet" because, whether it's a person or a food, the connotation of sweet is undeniably sweet.

Not that there aren't people who don't like sour—my

coauthor is a sour foods "freak," loves to suck on lemons. But for those of us who, whatever else we like to eat, love certain sweet foods or have a "sweet tooth," there has never been a reducing plan that truly satisfies you and is healthy enough over the long term. Of course, you won't be staying on the Sweet Diet for the long term, but for once you'll have the run of the entire candy store. At the end of a week or two you'll have basically satisfied your sweet tooth probably for the first time in your life, and you'll be more than happy to have just occasional sweets as you switch to the next BDS diet. All your life you've been told, "Don't eat sweets." Or, "You'd be better off if you'd eat less carbohydrates" (which almost every sweet food is high in). So, an occasional binge notwithstanding, if you're a sweet eater, you've had to hold back your whole life. That means that inside is a "person" who wants to devour sweet after sweet day after day, a "person" who has never been satisfied and thus isn't really happy even with an occasional hot fudge sundae or box of candy.

I'm going to give you a list of sweet foods and their approximate calorie count. You'll notice that many of them are fruits. Try as much as possible to build your Sweet-Tooth Diet around fruits. If you don't like this one or that one, try another you like somewhat, or one you haven't had before. You may find that with a little cream on your blackberries, they become a staple for you during this period.

Most of us with a sweet tooth have it for three reasons. First, sweets taste good. Some animals love nothing better than to find a piece of fruit. Give an ape a banana, and he couldn't be happier. But a second reason is that we're brought up on sweets. They are available, and they are sweet. Third, we tend to be brought up on manufactured sweets—candies and cakes and ice creams.

If you've been brought up on sweets and this has given you a sweet tooth, you can't change that. But what you can change to some extent is the sweets you eat. This diet will help you to do it, and will help you where calories are concerned.

However, unless the sweets you eat (and fruit helps a lot here) contain some proteins and fats, don't make them over 50 percent of your caloric intake. And here's something rather startling: Don't worry if you don't lose weight on the Sweet-Tooth Diet. The reason we have the Sweet-Tooth Diet is that during this period *you don't gain.* Even if you stay at the same weight you were from the previous BDS diet, you've accomplished something. Then you can go on to the next one, and lose some more. However, you may well lose a certain amount of weight, though not a lot, on the Sweet-Tooth Diet.

Like the other BDS diets, the Sweet-Tooth Diet works nicely both for those who have a sweet tooth and for those who don't. If you don't, you may not want to stay on it for two weeks—only a few days at most, where it becomes almost a dessert, a reward for the last diet or two you've been following. But if you do have a sweet tooth, it's an absolute necessity. When you come to your second cycle and to your Sweet-Tooth Diet again, you'll find that you're better able to eat enough sweets, but not as much as you have been eating, and also to eat healthier sweets.

Most Common Sweet Foods

	Calories
Apple juice (1 cup)	120
Apples (1 average)	60
Apricot (1 average)	19
Avocado (½ average)	188
Banana (1 average)	90
Beets (boiled, ½ cup)	31
Blackberries (1 serving)	39
Blueberries (1 serving)	42
Bread, raisin and cinnamon (1 slice)	65

Cakes

Angel food, no icing (1 serving)	265
Devil's food, with chocolate icing (1 serving)	375
White, with chocolate icing (1 serving)	350

Candies

Chocolate covered almonds (1 oz.)	163
Caramel, chocolate or vanilla (1 oz.)	115
Fudge, chocolate or vanilla (1 oz.)	115
Hard candy (1 oz.)	110
Coconut, chocolate covered (1 oz.)	125
Cantaloupe, fresh (½ melon)	56

Calories

Cereals

Branflakes (1 cup)	105
Cornflakes (1 cup)	98
Farina (1 cup)	105
Cherries, sweet (10 cherries)	50
Chocolate, semi-sweet chips (½ cup)	433
Coconut, fresh (1 piece)	160

Cookies

Animal crackers (1 oz.)	126
Chocolate (1 oz.)	128
Macaroon (1 oz.)	137
Oatmeal with raisins (1 oz.)	125
Sugar wafer (1 oz.)	139
Vanilla wafer (1 oz.)	133
Corn (boiled, 1 average ear)	72
Cornmeal, dry (½ cup)	220
Cranberries, fresh (½ cup)	25

Cream

Half and half (½ cup)	164
Sour (½ cup)	246
Whipping (½ cup)	360
Danish pastry (1 serving)	276
Dates (10 average)	222
Eggnog (1 cup)	250
Figs, fresh (1 small)	30
Fruit cocktail, canned (½ cup)	100
Gelatin dessert (½ cup)	70
Grapes, fresh (½ cup)	34
Grapefruit, fresh (½ average)	55
Gum, chewing (1 stick)	9

	Calories
Ice cream (½ cup)	135
Jams and preserves (1 oz.)	76

Milk

Whole (1 glass)	164
Skim (1 glass)	87
Buttermilk, cultured (1 glass)	85
Malted (1 glass)	246
Nectarines, fresh (1 average)	86
Orange juice, fresh (1 cup)	118
Oranges, fresh (1 average)	62
Pancakes, with syrup or jelly (2 average)	190
Peaches, fresh (1 average)	36
Peanut butter (1 tbsp.)	95
Pears, fresh (1 average)	102
Peas, green (boiled, ½ cup)	59

Pies

Apple (baked, 1 serving)	233
Cherry (baked, 1 serving)	285
Coconut custard (baked, 1 serving)	251
Pineapple, fresh (1 slice)	45
Plums, fresh (10 plums)	68
Prunes, dried (1 average)	15
Raisins, seedless (4 oz.)	330
Raspberries, fresh (½ cup)	38
Strawberries, fresh (½ cup)	27

Sugar

Brown (½ cup)	412
Granulated (½ cup)	387
Powdered (½ cup)	233
Waffles, with syrup or jelly (2 average)	485

20

The Six-Small-Meals-A-Day Diet

SOME YEARS AGO MUCH WAS MADE OF A LEADING SCI-entist's experiments on rats which showed that rodents who had six small meals a day lived noticeably longer than those who ate three large meals. I think there's something to this, partly because the kinds of "large" meals we humans eat are too large. However, the reason the BDS includes the half-a-dozen-or-so-small-meals-a-day diet is mainly because *you* can use it. If it increases your life-span, so much the better. What we're after here, though, is for it to decrease your waistline.

You can eat what you want on this diet, within this structure:

1. Balance the diet as much as possible between proteins, fats, and carbohydrates, as well as the different food groups, and, to the extent that your diet is unbalanced, of course go heavier on protein or low-cal salad-type foods.

2. Ease into the Six-Small-Meals-A-Day Diet. Not that most of you haven't been eating six meals a day, if one includes snacks (which really are small meals), but you haven't been doing it on purpose. So begin possibly with four or five or, on the other hand, seven or eight, then adjust it to six.

3. However you approach the Six-Small-Meals-a-Day Diet, the bottom line is that no more than 25 percent of your daily intake of calories should be expended on any one meal. You don't have to go one-sixth, one-sixth, one-sixth, and so forth. But if you expend a third or more of your calories on a single meal, you'll really be eating what amounts to one or two big meals and three or four small snacks, which isn't what the BDS Diet No. 5 is about. Also, you do have to count your calories a bit more closely on this diet than on some others. Because there's always the tendency to make those six small meals into six not-so-small ones. This is particularly true in the opening days of the diet. Once you get past those first two or three twenty-four hour periods, you'll be used to six small meals a day, so used to it that, as mentioned previously, you may want to extend the period for this diet to well over two weeks.

21

The No-Diet Diet

THERE IS SOMETHING IN ALMOST ALL OF US THAT abhors staying on a diet. That's part of what the Berkowitz Diet Switch is all about.

At the same time, most of us like—and need—to be given a structure to follow, in life as well as in eating. Yet even those among us who thrive best on a regular, even rigid, schedule, need a "vacation" from that schedule now and then.

The No-Diet Diet fills that need.

Except for calorie counting so that you maintain your weight loss (or even lose a few more pounds), the No-Diet Diet is completely without structure—you eat anything you want. Simultaneously, you are still within the structure of the BDS because you are doing this *purposefully* and for a *limited time.*

How I came upon this final diet for the BDS will tell you something of why you should come upon it.

I had kept my weight within a few pounds of what I wanted about 95 percent of the time for several years before I began testing it upon my patients. Their experience pretty much paralleled mine. The five other BDS diets got their weight down and, a huge amount of the time, kept it down. Yet why not nearly 100 percent of the time? One BDS ingredient was still missing.

I knew what was missing, but didn't know then how to make it into a diet. Because what was missing was that "vacation" from dieting. Since the BDS is a switching from diet to diet, this vacation wasn't needed as soon or as much compared to as when these people had tried to stick to a single diet. In some cases, of course, the BDS worked perfectly with the basic five. It can work with three. Two. One—in rare cases. Simply the switching seemed enough of a change from the same daily diet for a lot of people. Yet for others it wasn't. Sure, the diets they had tried before the BDS had begun to bore them after a few days or weeks, and on the Diet Switch it was the better part of a year before they even began to become the least bit bored.

Still, some of them *did* begin to find the BDS's continual variety a lack of variety—*precisely because the variety was continual.* Since I'd spent years finding the five best diets for them, and there really were no other diets to put them *on,* one day it occurred to me to tell them to go *off* their diets for a short time. Just a couple of days. It worked wonders.

And that was the creation of the No-Diet Diet.

Of course, you have to watch your calories. But you can eat what you want, six meals a day, high protein, lots of sweets, whatever you choose one day, whatever strikes your fancy the next. Usually, the first time around, at least, the No-Diet Diet shouldn't go for a full two weeks. Once you get used to it after several BDS cycles, you may be able to handle it for a couple of weeks. A few people have been able to handle it for years, because the BDS changed their eating habits and attitude toward overeating so much that they were actually able to maintain their weight on "no diet" at all. I analyzed what they ate, however, and found that what they were really doing was switching from one BDS diet to another, but over a matter of a couple of meals rather than a couple of weeks.

As long as diet switching is in the background, it doesn't always have to be in the foreground. Many people do best on a rather rigid and frequent switching pattern. But others, once they function for a while within the structure of the Diet Switch, discover that no matter which diet they are on or for how long, their weight is being kept where it belongs.

PART FOUR

The Berkowitz Personalized Diet Quiz

22

Ten Questions and Answers for a Slimmer You

AS YOU'VE JUST SEEN, THE BERKOWITZ DIET SWITCH IS made up of these six diets:

—High Protein Diet
—Bare Breakfast, Little Lunch, Deal-With-Dinner Diet
—Fill-up-on Salad-Or-Something-Similar Diet
—Sweet-Tooth Diet
—Six-Small-Meals-a-Day Diet
—No-Diet Diet

Now we want to find out which of the six diets are really for you—the individual you, with a very different body mechanism from mine or your cousin's or your friend Joe's. That is the object of this personalized diet quiz. Each question attempts to identify your basic food preference. For example, if you answer "A" to Question 1, this does not mean you usually *eat* meat or fish with baked potato or vegetable meals. It means that you prefer this meal over the other alternatives listed. (Choices A through F.) What we are getting at is your food *preference,* not your eating *habits.*

Each of the ten questions is followed by a brief explanation of what your answer means in general to you as a dieter. You will learn also whether your answer indicates that you would do well on one or more of the six diets, and possibly whether one of the diets may be wrong for you.

Here is what I am going to ask you to do: Wherever your answer to a question indicates that a specific diet is positive for you, put an "O" in the diet boxscore at the end of that question. Wherever your answer indicates that a diet has negative value for you, put an "X" in the diet boxscore.

If you feel that you may have misunderstood any question—or were not altogether honest with yourself about the answer—go back and reanswer. Remember there is no right or wrong answer. You're just asking yourself basic questions that I ask my own patients. The outcome, I believe, will help you to discover something about yourself that will finally make it really possible to get rid of that extra weight and keep it off.

QUESTION 1. CIRCLE THE ONE GROUP OF FOODS YOU WOULD GENERALLY PREFER TO EAT IF YOU WERE TO SIT DOWN TO A SINGLE MEAL, REGARDLESS OF THE TIME OF DAY: (SELECT FROM LETTERS A THROUGH F.)

A

Meat or fish
Potatoes or a
favorite vegetable
Dessert

B

A Sandwich
A couple of soft
drinks or beer

C

A couple of pieces
of cake, several
candy bars or a
sundae

D

An Italian or
Mexican dish
Bread and butter

E

Something
interesting that you
haven't eaten
before, prepared
well

F

An Omelet
Toast and bacon

Now, match the letter of your Food Preference with the corresponding letter below to find your own Food Profile. Remember to check the diet boxscore appropriately. (For example, if your food preference is "F"—an omelet and toast and bacon—you are a breakfast eater and in the diet boxscore you would put an "O" in the blank opposite every diet.)

A

You like a balanced meal. And your food tastes are probably pretty basic. Good candidates for High Protein, Fill-up-on-Salad, Bare Breakfast, and No-Diet diets.

B

You like to eat informally. Though there may be a couple of sandwiches in particular that you prefer, you want the option of eating what you like when you like. Positive for High Protein, Bare Breakfast, Fill-Up-On-Salad, Six-Small-Meals-A-Day, and No-Diet diets. Negative for Sweet Tooth Diet.

C

You have a "sweet tooth." Positive for Sweet and Bare Breakfast diets. Negative for Six-Meals-A-Day and No-Diet diets.

D

You like tasty, possibly spicy, foods. Positive for all diets, except negative for Six-Meals-A-Day diet.

E

Gourmet tendency. Positive for High Protein, Bare Breakfast, Fill-Up-On-Salad, and No-Diet diets. Negative for Sweet and Six-Meals-A-Day diets.

F

A breakfast eater. Positive for all diets.

DIET BOXSCORE

High Protein	_____	Sweet-Tooth	_____
Bare Breakfast	_____	Six-Small Meals	_____
Fill-Up-On-Salad	_____	No-Diet Diet	_____

QUESTION 2. CIRCLE ONE GROUP OF FOODS THAT YOU WOULD GENERALLY PREFER TO EAT *LEAST* IF YOU WERE TO HAVE A SINGLE MEAL OTHER THAN BREAKFAST: (SELECT FROM LETTERS A THROUGH F.)

A

A large salad

B

An omelet
Bacon or sausage

C

A sandwich
A soft drink or beer

D

Meat or fish
Potatoes or a
favorite vegetable
Dessert

E

A couple of pieces
of cake, several
candy bars, or a
sundae

F

Something
interesting that you
haven't eaten
before, prepared
well.

Match the letter below to your choice above. Remember to check the diet boxscore.

A

Positive for all diets, but possibly negative for Fill-Up-On-Salad.

B

Positive for all diets, especially the Bare Breakfast diet.

C

Positive for all diets, especially the Bare Breakfast diet.

D

Positive for all diets, especially the High Protein and Bare Breakfast diets.

E

Positive for all diets, especially the Sweet-Tooth Diet.

F

Positive for all diets, especially the Bare Breakfast, High Protein, Fill-Up-On-Salad Diets

DIET BOXSCORE

High Protein	_____	Sweet-Tooth	_____
Bare Breakfast	_____	Six-Small Meals	_____
Fill-Up-On-Salad	_____	No-Diet Diet	_____

QUESTION 3. AT WHAT TIME OF DAY DO YOU TEND TO OVEREAT MOST FREQUENTLY?

A
Late morning

B
Lunch

C
Midafternoon

D
Dinner

E
After dinner

F
Middle of the Night or Breakfast

Match the letter below to your choice above. Check the diet boxscore.

A

Small but solid breakfast may help. Tension or boredom might be a factor. Positive for all diets.

B

May not be getting enough protein early in the day. You might also have the habit of overeating "socially." Positive for all six diets.

C

Early meals may be insufficient. You may not be enjoying dinner itself enough. Positive for all six diets.

D

You and 50 million other Americans. Positive for all six diets.

E

You and 30 million Americans. All six diets should suit you.

F

This is a specialized but not uncommon overeating habit. Six-Small-Meals-A-Day is definitely helpful here, as are the other diets—with the exception of the No-Diet diet, which is negative for you in the first cycle of switching.

DIET BOXSCORE

High Protein	_____	Sweet-Tooth	_____
Bare Breakfast	_____	Six-Small Meals	_____
Fill-Up-On-Salad	_____	No-Diet Diet	_____

QUESTION 4. WHICH, IF ANY, OF THE FOLLOWING DIETS HAVE YOU USED MOST?

A
Low carbohydrate

B
Liquid

C
Calorie counting

D
A Concentrate-On-One-Food Diet

E
A group reducing plan

F
A "Crash" diet

Match the letter below to your choice above. Check the diet boxscore.

A
Positive for all diets, especially the High Protein.

B
Positive for all diets, especially Fill-Up-On-Salad.

C
Positive for all diets, especially the No-Diet

D
Positive for all diets, especially the Fill-Up-On-Salad and High Protein diets.

E
Positive for all diets except the No-Diet in the first switching cycle.

F
Positive for all diets, especially the Fill-Up-On-Salad and the High Protein.

DIET BOXSCORE

High Protein	————	Sweet-Tooth	————
Bare Breakfast	————	Six-Small-Meals	————
Fill-Up-On-Salad	————	No-Diet Diet	————

QUESTION 5. WHAT SINGLE EATING HABIT WOULD YOU SAY HAS CONTRIBUTED MOST TO YOUR OVER-WEIGHT?

A	**B**	**C**
Sweets	Snack foods	Too much dinner
D	**E**	**F**
Fast foods (sandwiches, pizzas, etc.)	Leftovers	"Nervous" eating

Match the letter below to your choice above. Check the diet boxscore.

A

You either have a sweet tooth or you don't. If you do, it's far better to work with it than to try and make it vanish away by magic. The Sweet Diet is tailored for you. All other diets—with the possible exception of the High Protein, which may be a negative for you—are answers.

B

This habit, on the other hand, can be frequently overcome. The best way to begin is the Six-Small-Meals-A-Day Diet, though all the other diets except the Sweet Diet will work.

C

Who among us doesn't eat too much dinner sometimes? Positive for all diets, especially the Bare Breakfast, Little Lunch, and Deal-With-Dinner Diet.

D

Positive for all diets. The later chapters in this book, where additional hints are given, will be especially helpful to you.

E

Positive for all diets, especially the Six-Small-Meals-A-Day Diet.

F

Positive for all diets. The later chapters in this book, where additional hints are given, will be especially helpful to you.

DIET BOXSCORE

High Protein	_____	Sweet-Tooth	_____
Bare Breakfast	_____	Six-Small Meals	_____
Fill-Up-On-Salad	_____	No-Diet Diet	_____

QUESTION 6. DO YOU OVEREAT MORE WHEN YOU ARE ALONE OR WITH OTHERS?

A
Alone

B
With others

Match the letter below to your choice above. Check the diet boxscore.

A

The two diets that might be question marks—or negative—are the Sweet-Tooth and the No-Diet Diet. The four others usually work wonders if you do more of your overeating alone.

B

The only diet that is a possible negative here is the Six-Small-Meals-A-Day. The reason is obvious: If you're already eating mainly with others and overweight, adding extra meals—even though small ones—will not strike the root of the problem.

DIET BOXSCORE

High Protein	_____	Sweet Tooth	_____
Bare Breakfast	_____	Six-Small-Meals	_____
Fill-Up-On-Salad	_____	No-Diet Diet	_____

QUESTION 7. WHEN YOU'VE BEEN OVERWEIGHT, ABOUT HOW MANY POUNDS HAS IT BEEN (CHECK MOST FREQUENT)?

A	**B**	**C**
15 pounds	25 pounds	35 pounds

D	**E**	
50 pounds	Over 65 pounds	

Match the letter below to your choice above. Check the diet boxscore.

A

Even if you weigh more now, if you've mainly been in this overweight bracket, it's minimal, and chances are you'll be down to your ideal weight through diet switching within a short time. All six diets "go."

B

More overweight people fall into this range than any other. Almost always this overweight arises because of one or two diet problems that one or two of the four or five diets on your Diet Switch will remedy. All six diets "go."

C

Nearly as frequent an overweight range. Once you lose the first 7 or 8 pounds, you'll find getting rid of the rest of your overweight relatively easy. Again, all diets "go."

D

This amount of weight should be lost in stages—taking off a few pounds or more with each diet to which you switch, holding at that level, then losing some more. All six diets are positive, but the No-Diet Diet should not be misused.

E

Same as D, except that the longer you have been this much overweight, the more gradually you should take it off. The body needs time to adjust, and you should feel elated by each step in the right direction. Sooner than you think, the steps will have become the main part of the journey.

DIET BOXSCORE

High Protein	_____	Sweet-Tooth	_____
Bare Breakfast	_____	Six-Small Meals	_____
Fill-Up-On-Salad	_____	No-Diet Diet	_____

QUESTION 8. HOW OVERWEIGHT ARE YOU RIGHT NOW?

A	B	C
15 pounds	25 pounds	35 pounds

D	E
50 pounds	Over 65 pounds

Match the letter below to your choice above. Check the diet boxscore.

A

It's minimal. Chances are you'll be down to your ideal weight through diet switching within a short time. All six diets "go."

B

More overweight people fall into this range than any other. Almost always this excess weight arises because of one or two diet problems that the Diet Switch will remedy unless you are coming down from a markedly higher weight. The High Protein is probably the best diet on which to begin, though all diets are positive.

C

Nearly as frequent an overweight range. Once you lose the first 7 or 8 pounds, you'll find getting rid of the rest of your overweight relatively easy. If you are coming down from a

D

This amount of weight should be lost in stages—taking off a few pounds or more with each diet to which you switch, holding at that level, then losing some more—unless you are

C (cont'd)
markedly higher weight, the High Protein is probably the best diet on which to begin, though all diets are positive.

D (cont'd)
coming down from a markedly higher weight. If you have come up to this rather rapidly from a lower weight, again the High Protein is the best diet to start with, and you should expect results in the first week, but not the first couple of days. Give your metabolism time to adjust. All diets are positive.

E
Like D, this amount of weight should be lost in stages, taking off a few pounds or more with each diet to which you switch, holding at that level, then losing some more. All diets are positive.

DIET BOXSCORE

High Protein	_____	Sweet-Tooth	_____
Bare Breakfast	_____	Six-Small-Meals	_____
Fill-Up-On-Salad	_____	No-Diet Diet	_____

QUESTION 9. WHAT PART OF YOUR LIFE HAVE YOU BEEN OVERWEIGHT?

A
Less than a year

B
Several years

C
Five to ten years

D
Closer to twenty years

E
Most of my life

F
Almost all my life, including most of my childhood

Match the letter below to your choice above. Check the diet boxscore.

A

Switching should bring you back to normal quickly. All diets positive.

B

Basically the same as A. All diets positive.

C

All diets positive, but you should probably begin on the High Protein, Fill-Up-On-Salad, Bare Breakfast, or Six-Small-Meals-A-Day diets.

D

All diets positive, but put the No-Diet last.

E

All diets positive, but watch carefully to see which should go longer than two weeks, which less than two weeks.

F

Same as above, except that on one or two of your switches you may need to keep the same weight rather than lose. This should not be discouraging. On the other diets you will lose weight.

DIET BOXSCORE

High Protein	_____	Sweet-Tooth	_____
Bare Breakfast	_____	Six-Small-Meals	_____
Fill-Up-On-Salad	_____	No-Diet Diet	_____

QUESTION 10. WHICH OF THE FOLLOWING IS YOUR STRONGEST FEELING AGAINST OVERWEIGHT

A
"It's unhealthy."

B
"It makes me less attractive to others."

C
"I don't like to look at myself."

D
"I feel guilty about it."

Match the letter below to your choice above. Check the diet boxscore.

A

All diets positive, especially High Protein and Fill-Up-On-Salad.

B

All diets positive, but try to have fewer meals alone.

C

All diets positive, and Six-Small-Meals-A-Day may be especially helpful here.

D

All diets positive, but watch yourself carefully on the No-Diet Diet.

DIET BOXSCORE

High Protein	_____	Sweet-Tooth	_____
Bare Breakfast	_____	Six-Small-Meals	_____
Fill-Up-On-Salad	_____	No-Diet Diet	_____

23

Adding Up
Your Answers

NOW LET'S SEE WHAT YOUR ANSWERS ADD UP TO IN
starting you off on the Berkowitz Diet Switch.

When I am asking the questions in person, my assumption is that at least five, maybe all six, of the diets will be
suitable. Sometimes, though, an individual's answers reveal
that not one, but two, diets are negative. Whatever the
count, this is what you do:

1. Go through your answers, and where your answer
indicated that a diet is positive for you, put an O under that
diet in the list at the end of this chapter. Where your answer
indicated that a diet has negative value for you, put an X
under that diet.

2. For each of the six diets subtract the number of X's from the number of O's. This will tell you how many of the six BDS diets you'll use. It may indicate also the order in which you use them.

First, any diet that you have marked with more X's than O's—or even with as many as two X's—should be eliminated, at least the first time around.

Second, this will leave you with four, probably five, possibly all six diets. The diet you should go on first is the one with the most O's. The diet you should go on next is the one with the second most O's. And so on.

It is possible that you may have, say, three O's under the name of one diet and an X. *You should count that as two O's.* It is also possible that you may have the same number of O's for more than one diet. In that case, follow the order of the diets as they are listed. Another way of putting it is: In figuring out where to begin and where to go from there, begin with the six diets as I have listed them, then change the order according to the most O's.

QUIZ SCORE SHEET

HIGH PROTEIN DIET

Quiz Score: _____

BARE BREAKFAST, LITTLE LUNCH, AND DEAL-WITH-DINNER DIET

Quiz Score: _____

FILL-UP-ON-SALAD OR SOMETHING-SIMILAR DIET

Quiz Score: _____

SWEET-TOOTH DIET

Quiz Score: _____

SIX-SMALL-MEALS-A-DAY DIET

Quiz Score: _____

NO-DIET DIET

Quiz Score: _____

24

Losing Weight

THIRTY-FIVE HUNDRED CALORIES, MORE OR LESS, MAKE up a pound. If you want to lose several pounds a week on the BDS, you'll have to cut down the calories you are eating by about 1,500 or 1,800 a day.

It's not all that easy to figure out how many calories you've been taking in. And certainly you don't want to overeat for another week or two to find out! Besides, most people, when they make a count, underestimate. Another problem is you can't go strictly by the number of calories needed to maintain the right weight for a person of your sex and build. If you're 45 pounds overweight, for example, you're taking in a lot more calories than a person 15 pounds overweight. To try and cut off all those extra calories in one fell swoop is unrealistic. (To determine your approximate daily caloric needs, see tables in Appendix C.)

The most sensible way to lose a reasonable, healthy amount of weight each week is this: If you're under 25 pounds overweight, go by the basic caloric needs for your build and sex. But if you're heavier than that, add at least several hundred more calories daily to that intake. Then test it out. If you lose a few pounds your first week, you'll know you figured it about right. If you lose less than that, then decrease your calorie intake slightly. If by any chance you lose more, though I know you'll be happy about it, it's best to add some calories. Weight taken off slowly but surely is more permanently gone than "crash" reducing. Remember: the BDS is a way of life, a way of eating, if you will, that is to yours from here on out. So take your time and enjoy yourself while going about it.

Also, though we'll stress this a number of other times, no matter which of the diets you're on, you should have something from each of the major food groups at least every couple or three days. Foods are usually classified according to proteins, fats, carbohydrates, vitamins and minerals. Food "groups"—those things nature meant us to have— are classified as dairy products, meat, fish, eggs, and poultry, cereal and whole grains, green and yellow vegetables, and fruits. For optimal health don't ignore any one of them for too long a time.

In Appendix C you will find charts for men and for women giving you a general idea of your caloric needs according to height and body type. Appendix D tells you about carbohydrates, fats, and proteins in most common foods, and signals which of the six BDS diets includes each particular food.

25

What You Should Know About The Berkowitz Diet Switch

NOW THAT YOU'VE SEEN WHAT THE SIX ACTUAL DIETS are like, and taken the quiz, there's something you should know. The *switching* of the diets is the key to the originality and success of the BDS. The diets are not in themselves revolutionary. By the same token, they all have one thing in common: they are basically balanced.

We have gone into the psychological and motivational reasons why other diets succeed for awhile and then almost surely fail. The *metabolic* or physiological reason the failure is so sudden and complete is that when you go *off* a diet that is basically unbalanced, as most of them are, the body is just lying in wait for what you haven't been giving it. It takes those new kinds of calories—carbohydrates, in particular—and turns them into fat faster than you can say, "I've gained ten pounds!"

The low-carbohydrate or almost-no-carbohydrate diet type is a good example. You lose weight when you take in only proteins and fats because of the catalytic process between the two—they tend to burn each other up more. But the minute you go off that diet and start eating those carbohydrates, zoom!

The BDS avoids this, even on the most "extreme" of our diets, by making sure that they are, all in all, metabolically balanced. I wouldn't recommend a diet that wasn't, anyway. It isn't healthy.

Your food intake does not have to be balanced, as you'll see, every day. Over the course of a couple or three or four days, and certainly a couple or three or four weeks, it does have to be. Not only because that's healthy, but because you will switch to another diet, and, if there were an imbalance, nature will out and pounds will result.

So, though the BDS switches have been scientifically tested, they are more behaviorally or psychologically oriented than metabolically—because metabolically you can move freely from one BDS diet to another without any problem. We asked the ten key questions principally so that you can start on the diet that gives you the best psychological start, and move in a pattern that makes the most sense for you as an individual.

Summing up, the BDS diets can be switched without a problem, as far as your physiology is concerned, because they are all basically balanced. And balance within a diet is a prime nutritional principle that has been established for decades. The BDS did not discover this principle, but instead uses it as a cornerstone upon which to build.

26

Should You Try The Berkowitz Diet Switch?

THERE ARE A FEW SMALL SEGMENTS OF THE POPULA-tion who should not go on the Berkowitz Diet Switch, mainly for medical reasons. The following questions will indicate whether you are in one of them:

1. Do you have an allergy to one or more food groups that is quite severe?

2. Do you have a serious chronic condition, such as di-abetes or heart trouble?

3. Are you on some kind of permanent prescription med-ication?

4. Are you more than 75 pounds overweight?

5. Are you over 70 years of age and in good health?

The question on allergies is more important than most people realize. Some of us are allergic to foods without knowing it. We have frequent indigestion, headaches, diarrhea, even a feeling of fatigue and depression, and we attribute it to a virus or psychological causes instead of the very frequent cause of food allergy. However, one of the "extras" of the Berkowitz Diet Switch is that because you will move from one different food "group" to another for a goodly amount of time, you may discover the allergy you didn't know you had because you will be suddenly free of those minor complaints. If you do discover this, by the way, simply eliminate the diet that gives you the discomfort. If your allergies are so severe, though, that you know what they are, and simply can't eat this food or that without actually getting sick, you still *may* be able to make the BDS work for you. But you have to eliminate whatever groups contain those allergy-producing foods at the start. If that leaves at least three diets to switch between, fine.

Obviously, a serious chronic condition—even though controlled by a physician—means that you must check with your physician before changing your eating habits. It might be a good idea to check with your physician before you go on *any* diet. The fact is, however, that most people eat with so little discretion much of the time that the chances are 99 out of 100 the BDS will be a vast improvement.

What is true for a chronic medical condition is true also for the taking of medication, whether for medical or psychological reasons. Prescription drugs are given by prescription for a reason. They contain one or more strong chemicals, and certain foods or beverages may be contraindicated. So again, if you are on pills regularly, consult your doctor before you embark on this or any other diet. However, another "plus" of the BDS is that people who have been taking prescription drugs regularly *not* for a chronic medical condition often find that the Berkowitz Diet Switch enables them to get off these pills. I've known of a number of men and women, for instance, who used prescription tranquilizers heavily. Yet they gained enough energy, excitement, and self-esteem through their successful diet-switching to throw away their pills.

As for being more than 75 pounds overweight, the BDS is *probably* for you, *but only after you see your doctor.* I've had a number of people this heavy, several even much heavier, in fact, who actually got down to their normal weight on the switching plan. Still, 75 pounds or more is not merely overweight, it is obesity, and thus it is a medical problem before it is a dietary one. You have to make sure that being overweight doesn't come from some cause other than eating. The chances are it doesn't. Even so, it is still a medical problem to be checked out with your physician before beginning the BDS.

So if you answered "yes" to any of the five questions at the beginning of this chapter, you may be one of that small minority who shouldn't try the BDS. What about the fifth question? You *can*—and I've had people do it successfully—be over 70 and in good health and overweight and adopt the BDS. But generally I don't encourage it, and I'll tell you why. If you're over 70 and in good health, even though you're overweight, you've been doing something right. There's an integrity to each individual's human physical constitution, and the chances are that if you have gotten to three score and ten and aren't suffering any serious health problems, you should stay as sweet as you are. Even if that means that you eat a lot of sweets!

There *is* one exception. If you've gained the weight very recently, it should be taken off.

The second qualifier, before we go to the six diets, is that I advise taking a good multiple vitamin pill. Even though the six BDS diets are balanced, a little insurance doesn't hurt. I agree to an extent with the natural foods people who feel that we don't get enough vitamins in our diet, particularly E and C. However, don't push a good thing. Taking too much of vitamins A and D, for example, can create serious problems. But a single good multivitamin capsule a day or, better, three smaller complete vitamins taken with meals so that their absorption is increased by the digestive process, is a good idea for all of us.

27

You Already Have Hundreds of Menus!

BEFORE THEY EMBARKED ON DIET SWITCHING, A NUM-ber of people asked me, "Where are the menus?" My answer: "You already have hundreds of menus."

THE BIGGEST SPECIFIC REASON WHY ALL OTHER DIETS HAVE FAILED YOU BEFORE IS BECAUSE THEY GIVE YOU MENUS AND FOOD LISTS.

The reason that the Diet Switch succeeds is that it *understands* that you *already* know *what* you *like* to eat and *how* you *like* to eat it.

There are two main things that are destructive about giving people menus or advice on what to eat.

The first reason, to go back to what we talked about at

the very beginning, is that menus or controlled groups of food from which you have to choose soon become boring and oppressive. In the beginning they are kind of fun, and that's why in the beginning you lose weight on just about every new diet. But not too long after the beginning, you begin to gain the weight back, and that's the end of that diet. And the biggest reason is that here are these same menus or combinations of foods staring you in the face day after day, and if you're in your right mind, you can't see a whole lifetime of that.

A second big reason why menus and food lists are destructive where beating overweight is concerned is that THEY AREN'T YOUR MENUS!

How dare someone else, no matter what kind of an expert he thinks he is, tell you that you'll have to like to eat this and you'll have to like to eat that, or else you won't be slim? What unrealistic pomposity!

Of course, the diets you've tried that have failed you didn't mean to be pompous. They meant to be helpful. But because they were unrealistic, because they didn't understand what overweight is really all about, they thought that "somehow" you could learn to like the medicine they were giving you if it was a little sugar-coated. Well, let's be straight with one another: Most of you have been periodically overweight for twenty years or more—even if you're a teenager, you've probably been overweight most of your life. Do you know how many days ten years of overweight is? It's *thousands*. And the point isn't that it's so terrible to have been overweight that many days. The point is that we're overweight because we eat too much, and if we've been eating too much of this and too much of that for thousands of days, which means *tens of thousands* of meals, we damn well know what we like to eat by now!

And no one is going to be able to have us suddenly like something else just because it will fit into that individual's particular plan for taking off pounds.

In the chapter following this I'm going to give you probably the most exact instructions you've ever had—instructions that even a young school child can understand—on how and when to switch diets. The reason I make the instructions so explicit is because diet switching is a new idea, and no matter how superintelligent you are, it's better to spell it out step by step. But I would never insult your intelligence and your individuality by telling you what you like to eat.

The ultimate reason other diets have failed you—and this is what burdens you with their little lists and mundane menus—is that they don't really value or know how to cope with individual tastes and needs *and* still deal with overweight. Frankly, I think they unwittingly insult your intelligence, too. Even a fourth-grader can count calories. So why do *they* have to count them up *for you?* The only possible reason can be that they want to make absolutely sure that you eat what *they* want you to eat, not what *you* want to eat, because they know that if you don't do exactly as they say, their diet won't work. It's like the teacher who can teach only one way and says to the students, "Do it my way—or you won't learn."

Well, if you're able and interested enough to read a book—and since you're reading these words, you *are*— you're definitely intelligent enough to add 25 and 270 and 33.

But that 25, that 270, and that 33 isn't a uniform you have to wear. It's a whole closet filled with all the clothes you yourself have chosen, and each day you can pretty much put on what you want.

That this unusual freedom is built into our Diet Switch is crucial to why it works and works permanently. Yes, I've given you some examples of sample small breakfasts, or opened you up hopefully to some sweet foods that are lower in calories and healthier for you than some of the sweets you've been eating, and "lists" like that.

But how in the world could I give you suggested meals or menus or combinations of foods for each of the six diets? It would be patently ridiculous. And the reason it's ridiculous is, you'll see, what makes these six diets so glorious to eat.

Take the No-Diet Diet, for an opener. You can eat *anything,* just as long as there's a certain healthy balance. And who doesn't want to stay healthy? That's one of the big reasons you want to lose weight.

But let's go further. It's pretty obvious that you can eat virtually the same thing on the Six-Small-Meals-A-Day Diet as you do on the High Protein Diet and the Bare Breakfast, Little Lunch, and Deal-With-Dinner Diet!

My coauthor's two favorite meals, for instance, are a seafood dinner with baked potato or a huge salad with a couple of kinds of dressing and some liberally sprinkled herbs and spices. He can make that work for almost any of the six diets, and that's one of the reasons why he's been able to maintain a weight of 145 pounds on his average height-average frame about 90 percent of his life. Once in a while he does go 10 or 20 pounds too heavy, by staying on the

Fill-Up-On-Salad Diet too long and adding too much sea-food to it, but switching brings him back to his normal weight within a short time. If I had recommended to Paul that he suddenly start eating avocados or eggs, it wouldn't work. Not only would he probably gain weight instead of lose it, but he'd be sick to his stomach. It would be like trying to make a vegetarian out of him. Or trying to make a meat-eater out of a vegetarian.

I have a healthy respect for you. And I have a healthy respect for why people overeat.

Most of us—and every one of us reading this book, as well as its author—wake up each morning and go to bed each night with the knowledge that, as that beer commercial goes, you only go around once in life. We want everything. We want the whole run of the candy store.

Diet switching gives you the run of the candy store—your particular candy store. What it also does, which is our key, is to tell you how to handle the candy store.

But won't you want to eat everything in a candy store? No.

Do you know why you have that urge so often? It's because without a plan, a scientific method of diet switching, you don't know how to handle eating what you like. That's perfectly natural. Animals in the jungle don't either. The difference is that because they have to expend so much energy to get their food and sometimes don't get enough, they can afford to gorge themselves when they get in their particular candy store.

And the other side of that coin is that the diets you've been given throughout the years have told you that, basically, your particular candy store is a no-no. Which means, in a sense, that what you *want* and what you *are* is a no-no. Diets like that are doomed to failure. All they create after the first few weeks or months is an uncontrollable urge to get into that candy store and eat every last chocolate meltaway.

Once you're living in the candy store—or the lobster store or the chili store or whatever your particular "store" is on diet switching—you won't feel that uncontrollable urge. You have everything available. Emotionally, you can afford to pick and choose. Who really wants to gorge themselves at every meal? It doesn't feel good. It doesn't let you enjoy the next meal as much. It makes you fat, and it makes you unhealthy.

BUT IT'S JUST AS UNHEALTHY TO HAVE THAT CANDY STORE—TO HAVE WHAT YOU LIKE TO EAT—TAKEN AWAY FROM YOU.

Oh, you'll overeat, you'll even gorge yourself now and then. Big deal. That's part of what being human is all about.

What the Diet Switch enables you to do is to overeat, and then go right back to eating what you like sensibly.

Diet switching looks at you as both the horse and the horseman. The animal in you, the appetite in you, can run as fast as you want, as far as you want, wherever you want.

But the nonanimal part of you will always be in the saddle, always finally in control, always holding the reins.

28

Exactly When
to Switch

YOU SWITCH FROM ONE DIET TO THE NEXT WHEN YOU
have lost a certain amount of weight.

If you have not lost that amount of weight *within two weeks,* you *switch* anyway.

Once in a while you will *not* lose weight on a particular diet. In that case, switch at once—*unless* the weight gain occurs in the first *thirty-six* hours. If you gain weight on a diet, *do not include* that diet in your *next* switching cycle.

Do *not* weigh yourself more than once a day. Preferably, weigh yourself *every forty-eight hours,* or even *every three days.* Weigh yourself *at approximately the same time* during the day or evening whenever you do get on the scale.

Now . . .

IF YOU ARE LESS THAN
15 POUNDS OVERWEIGHT

—SWITCH FROM YOUR FIRST DIET TO YOUR SECOND ONCE YOU LOSE 4 POUNDS.

—SWITCH FROM YOUR SECOND DIET TO YOUR THIRD ONCE YOU LOSE ANOTHER 3 POUNDS.

—SWITCH FROM YOUR THIRD DIET TO YOUR FOURTH ONCE YOU LOSE ANOTHER 2 POUNDS.

—SWITCH FROM YOUR FOURTH DIET TO YOUR FIFTH ONCE YOU LOSE ANOTHER 2 POUNDS.

—SWITCH FROM YOUR FIFTH DIET TO YOUR SIXTH ONCE YOU LOSE ANOTHER 2 POUNDS.

—SWITCH FROM YOUR SIXTH DIET TO YOUR FIRST ONCE YOU LOSE ANOTHER 2 POUNDS.

If you are on only four or five of the diets instead of six, simply start the cycle again.

If you have not lost all the weight you want to lose by the end of the first cycle, simply repeat it, but this time *eliminate* the diet on which you lost the *least weight.*

If you lose *all* of your overweight *before* completing the cycle, complete it anyway. *Repeat* the cycle exactly as is a second time. If you *maintain* your weight loss, keep repeating the cycle exactly as is. *However,* if you put on 3 pounds or more, *reverse* the cycle. Or, if at any time, though your weight loss is still maintained, the cycle begins to bore you even in the least, *reverse* the cycle.

Once you have completed three cycles of diet switching,

you can rearrange the four or five or six diets *according to your own inclination.* But if you gain 3 pounds or more, go back to your original cycle according to your answers to the ten questions.

IF YOU ARE 16-25 POUNDS OVERWEIGHT,
YOU SHOULD LOSE THIS OVERWEIGHT
IN **TWO** CYCLES, NOT ONE.

FIRST CYCLE:
—SWITCH FROM YOUR FIRST DIET TO YOUR SECOND ONCE YOU LOSE 4 POUNDS.
—SWITCH FROM YOUR SECOND DIET TO YOUR THIRD ONCE YOU LOSE ANOTHER 3 POUNDS.
—SWITCH FROM YOUR THIRD DIET TO YOUR FOURTH ONCE YOU LOSE ANOTHER 2 POUNDS.
—SWITCH FROM YOUR FOURTH DIET TO YOUR FIFTH ONCE YOU LOSE ANOTHER 2 POUNDS.
—SWITCH FROM YOUR FIFTH DIET TO YOUR SIXTH ONCE YOU LOSE ANOTHER 2 POUNDS.
—SWITCH FROM YOUR SIXTH DIET TO YOUR FIRST ONCE YOU LOSE ANOTHER 2 POUNDS.

SECOND CYCLE:
—SWITCH FROM YOUR FIRST DIET TO YOUR SECOND ONCE YOU LOSE ANOTHER 3 POUNDS.
—SWITCH FROM YOUR SECOND DIET TO YOUR THIRD ONCE YOU LOSE ANOTHER 2 POUNDS.
—SWITCH FROM YOUR THIRD DIET TO YOUR FOURTH ONCE YOU LOSE ANOTHER 2 POUNDS.

—SWITCH FROM YOUR FOURTH DIET TO YOUR FIFTH ONCE
   YOU LOSE 1 POUND.
—SWITCH FROM YOUR FIFTH DIET TO YOUR SIXTH ONCE YOU
   LOSE 1 POUND.
—SWITCH FROM YOUR SIXTH DIET TO YOUR FIRST ONCE YOU
   LOSE 1 POUND.

If you are on only four or five of the diets instead of six,
simply start the cycle again.

If you have not lost all the weight you want to by the end
of the cycles, simply repeat—but this time *eliminate* the diet
on which you lost the *least weight*.

If you lose *all* of your overweight *before* completing the
cycles, complete them anyway. *Repeat* the cycles exactly
as is. If you *maintain* your weight loss, keep repeating exactly as is. However, if you put on 3 pounds or more,
reverse the cycle. Or, if at any time, though your weight
loss is still maintained, the cycle begins to bore you *even*
in the least, *reverse* the cycle.

Once you have completed *three* cycles of diet switching,
you can rearrange the four or five or six diets *according to
your own inclination.* But if you gain 3 pounds or more, *go
back to* your original cycle according to your answers to the
ten questions.

IF YOU ARE 26-35 POUNDS OVERWEIGHT,
YOU SHOULD LOSE THIS OVERWEIGHT
IN **THREE** CYCLES.

FIRST CYCLE:
—SWITCH FROM YOUR FIRST DIET TO YOUR SECOND ONCE
   YOU LOSE 4 POUNDS.

—SWITCH FROM YOUR SECOND DIET TO YOUR THIRD ONCE YOU LOSE ANOTHER 3 POUNDS.

—SWITCH FROM YOUR THIRD DIET TO YOUR FOURTH ONCE YOU LOSE ANOTHER 2 POUNDS.

—SWITCH FROM YOUR FOURTH DIET TO YOUR FIFTH ONCE YOU LOSE ANOTHER 2 POUNDS.

—SWITCH FROM YOUR FIFTH DIET TO YOUR SIXTH ONCE YOU LOSE ANOTHER 2 POUNDS.

—SWITCH FROM YOUR SIXTH DIET TO YOUR FIRST ONCE YOU LOSE ANOTHER 2 POUNDS.

SECOND CYCLE:

—SWITCH FROM YOUR FIRST DIET TO YOUR SECOND ONCE YOU LOSE 3 POUNDS.

—SWITCH FROM YOUR SECOND DIET TO YOUR THIRD ONCE YOU LOSE ANOTHER 2 POUNDS.

—SWITCH FROM YOUR THIRD DIET TO YOUR FOURTH ONCE YOU LOSE ANOTHER 2 POUNDS.

—SWITCH FROM YOUR FOURTH DIET TO YOUR FIFTH ONCE YOU LOSE 1 POUND.

—SWITCH FROM YOUR FIFTH DIET TO YOUR SIXTH ONCE YOU LOSE 1 POUND.

—SWITCH FROM YOUR SIXTH DIET TO YOUR FIRST ONCE YOU LOSE 1 POUND.

THIRD CYCLE:

—SWITCH FROM YOUR FIRST DIET TO YOUR SECOND ONCE YOU LOSE 3 POUNDS.

—SWITCH FROM YOUR SECOND DIET TO YOUR THIRD ONCE YOU LOSE ANOTHER 2 POUNDS.

—SWITCH FROM YOUR THIRD DIET TO YOUR FOURTH ONCE YOU LOSE ANOTHER 2 POUNDS.

—SWITCH FROM YOUR FOURTH DIET TO YOUR FIFTH ONCE YOU LOSE 1 POUND.

—SWITCH FROM YOUR FIFTH DIET TO YOUR SIXTH ONCE YOU LOSE 1 POUND.

—SWITCH FROM YOUR SIXTH DIET TO YOUR FIRST ONCE YOU LOSE 1 POUND.

If you are on only four or five of the diets instead of six, simply start the cycle again.

If you have not lost all the weight that you want to by the end of the cycles, simply repeat—but this time *eliminate* the diet on which you lost the *least weight.*

If you lose *all* of your overweight *before* completing the cycles, complete them anyway. *Repeat* the cycles exactly as is. If you *maintain* your weight loss, keep repeating exactly as is. However, if you put on 3 pounds or more, *reverse* the cycle. Or, if at any time, though your weight loss is still maintained, the cycle begins to *bore* you even in the least, *reverse* the cycle.

Once you have completed *three* cycles of diet-switching, you can *rearrange* the four or five or six diets *according to your own feeling.* But if you gain 3 pounds or more, *go back to* your original cycle according to your answers to the ten questions.

IF YOU ARE 36-50 POUNDS OVERWEIGHT,
YOU SHOULD LOSE THIS OVERWEIGHT
IN **FOUR** CYCLES.

FIRST CYCLE:

—SWITCH FROM YOUR FIRST DIET TO YOUR SECOND ONCE YOU LOSE 4 POUNDS.

—SWITCH FROM YOUR SECOND DIET TO YOUR THIRD ONCE YOU LOSE ANOTHER 3 POUNDS.

—SWITCH FROM YOUR THIRD DIET TO YOUR FOURTH ONCE YOU LOSE ANOTHER 2 POUNDS.

—SWITCH FROM YOUR FOURTH DIET TO YOUR FIFTH ONCE YOU LOSE ANOTHER 2 POUNDS.

—SWITCH FROM YOUR FIFTH DIET TO YOUR SIXTH ONCE YOU LOSE ANOTHER 2 POUNDS.

—SWITCH FROM YOUR SIXTH DIET TO YOUR FIRST ONCE YOU LOSE ANOTHER 2 POUNDS.

SECOND CYCLE:

—SWITCH FROM YOUR FIRST DIET TO YOUR SECOND ONCE YOU LOSE 4 POUNDS.

—SWITCH FROM YOUR SECOND DIET TO YOUR THIRD ONCE YOU LOSE 3 POUNDS.

—SWITCH FROM YOUR THIRD DIET TO YOUR FOURTH ONCE YOU LOSE ANOTHER 2 POUNDS

—SWITCH FROM YOUR FOURTH DIET TO YOUR FIFTH ONCE YOU LOSE ANOTHER 2 POUNDS.

—SWITCH FROM YOUR FIFTH DIET TO YOUR SIXTH ONCE YOU LOSE ANOTHER 2 POUNDS.

—SWITCH FROM YOUR SIXTH DIET TO YOUR FIRST ONCE YOU LOSE ANOTHER 2 POUNDS.

THIRD CYCLE:

—SWITCH FROM YOUR FIRST DIET TO YOUR SECOND ONCE YOU LOSE 3 POUNDS.

—SWITCH FROM YOUR SECOND DIET TO YOUR THIRD ONCE YOU LOSE ANOTHER 2 POUNDS.

—SWITCH FROM THIRD DIET TO YOUR FOURTH ONCE YOU LOSE ANOTHER 2 POUNDS.

—SWITCH FROM YOUR FOURTH DIET TO YOUR FIFTH ONCE
YOU LOSE 1 POUND.

—SWITCH FROM YOUR FIFTH DIET TO YOUR SIXTH ONCE YOU
LOSE 1 POUND.

—SWITCH FROM YOUR SIXTH DIET TO YOUR FIRST ONCE YOU
LOSE 1 POUND.

FOURTH CYCLE:

—SWITCH FROM YOUR FIRST DIET TO YOUR SECOND ONCE
YOU LOSE 3 POUNDS.

—SWITCH FROM YOUR SECOND DIET TO YOUR THIRD ONCE
YOU LOSE ANOTHER 2 POUNDS.

—SWITCH FROM YOUR THIRD DIET TO YOUR FOURTH ONCE
YOU LOSE ANOTHER 2 POUNDS.

—SWITCH FROM YOUR FOURTH DIET TO YOUR FIFTH ONCE
YOU LOSE 1 POUND.

—SWITCH FROM YOUR FIFTH DIET TO YOUR SIXTH ONCE YOU
LOSE 1 POUND.

—SWITCH FROM YOUR SIXTH DIET TO YOUR FIRST ONCE YOU
LOSE 1 POUND.

If you are on only four or five of the diets instead of six,
simply start the cycle again.

If you have not lost all the weight that you want to by
the end of the cycles, simply repeat—but this time *eliminate*
the diet on which you lost the *least weight.*

If you lose *all* of your overweight *before* completing the
cycles, complete them anyway. *Repeat* the cycles exactly
as is. If you *maintain* your weight loss, keep repeating exactly as is. However, if you put on 3 pounds or more,
reverse the cycle. Or, if at any time, though your weight

loss is still maintained, the cycle begins to *bore* you even in the *least, reverse* the cycle.

Once you have completed *three* cycles of diet switching, you can *rearrange* the four or five or six diets *according to your own feeling*. But if you gain 3 pounds or more, *go back to* your original cycle according to your answers to the ten questions.

IF YOU ARE 51-65 POUNDS OVERWEIGHT,
YOU SHOULD LOSE THIS OVERWEIGHT
IN **FIVE** CYCLES.

FIRST CYCLE:

—SWITCH FROM YOUR FIRST DIET TO YOUR SECOND ONCE YOU LOSE 4 POUNDS.

—SWITCH FROM YOUR SECOND DIET TO YOUR THIRD ONCE YOU LOSE ANOTHER 3 POUNDS.

—SWITCH FROM YOUR THIRD DIET TO YOUR FOURTH ONCE YOU LOSE ANOTHER 2 POUNDS.

SWITCH FROM YOUR FOURTH DIET TO YOUR FIFTH ONCE YOU LOSE ANOTHER 2 POUNDS.

—SWITCH FROM YOUR FIFTH DIET TO YOUR SIXTH ONCE YOU LOSE ANOTHER 2 POUNDS.

—SWITCH FROM YOUR SIXTH DIET TO YOUR FIRST ONCE YOU LOSE ANOTHER 2 POUNDS.

SECOND CYCLE:

—SWITCH FROM YOUR FIRST DIET TO YOUR SECOND ONCE YOU LOSE 4 POUNDS.

—SWITCH FROM YOUR SECOND DIET TO YOUR THIRD ONCE YOU LOSE ANOTHER 3 POUNDS.

—SWITCH FROM YOUR THIRD DIET TO YOUR FOURTH ONCE YOU LOSE ANOTHER 2 POUNDS.

—SWITCH FROM YOUR FOURTH DIET TO YOUR FIFTH ONCE YOU LOSE ANOTHER 2 POUNDS.

—SWITCH FROM YOUR FIFTH DIET TO YOUR SIXTH ONCE YOU LOSE ANOTHER 2 POUNDS.

—SWITCH FROM YOUR SIXTH DIET TO YOUR FIRST ONCE YOU LOSE ANOTHER 2 POUNDS.

THIRD CYCLE:

—SWITCH FROM YOUR FIRST DIET TO YOUR SECOND ONCE YOU LOSE 4 POUNDS.

—SWITCH FROM YOUR SECOND DIET TO YOUR THIRD ONCE YOU LOSE ANOTHER 3 POUNDS.

—SWITCH FROM YOUR THIRD DIET TO YOUR FOURTH ONCE YOU LOSE ANOTHER 2 POUNDS.

—SWITCH FROM YOUR FOURTH DIET TO YOUR FIFTH ONCE YOU LOSE ANOTHER 2 POUNDS.

—SWITCH FROM YOUR FIFTH DIET TO YOUR SIXTH ONCE YOU LOSE ANOTHER 2 POUNDS.

—SWITCH FROM YOUR SIXTH DIET TO YOUR FIRST ONCE YOU LOSE ANOTHER 2 POUNDS.

FOURTH CYCLE:

—SWITCH FROM YOUR FIRST DIET TO YOUR SECOND ONCE YOU LOSE 3 POUNDS.

—SWITCH FROM YOUR SECOND DIET TO YOUR THIRD ONCE YOU LOSE ANOTHER 2 POUNDS.

—SWITCH FROM YOUR THIRD DIET TO YOUR FOURTH ONCE YOU LOSE ANOTHER 2 POUNDS.

—SWITCH FROM YOUR FOURTH DIET TO YOUR FIFTH ONCE YOU LOSE 1 POUND.

—SWITCH FROM YOUR FIFTH DIET TO YOUR SIXTH ONCE YOU LOSE 1 POUND.

—SWITCH FROM YOUR SIXTH DIET TO YOUR FIRST ONCE YOU LOSE 1 POUND.

FIFTH CYCLE:

—SWITCH FROM YOUR FIRST DIET TO YOUR SECOND ONCE YOU LOSE 3 POUNDS.

—SWITCH FROM YOUR SECOND DIET TO YOUR THIRD ONCE YOU LOSE ANOTHER 2 POUNDS.

—SWITCH FROM YOUR THIRD DIET TO YOUR FOURTH ONCE YOU LOSE ANOTHER 2 POUNDS.

—SWITCH FROM YOUR FOURTH DIET TO YOUR FIFTH ONCE YOU LOSE 1 POUND.

—SWITCH FROM YOUR FIFTH DIET TO YOUR SIXTH ONCE YOU LOSE 1 POUND.

—SWITCH FROM YOUR SIXTH DIET TO YOUR FIRST ONCE YOU LOSE 1 POUND.

If you are on only four or five of the diets instead of six, simply start the cycle again.

If you have not lost all the weight that you want to by the end of the cycles, simply repeat—but this time *eliminate* the diet on which you lost the *least weight.*

If you lose *all* of your overweight *before* completing the cycles, complete them anyway. *Repeat* the cycles exactly as is. If you *maintain* your weight loss, keep repeating exactly as is. *However,* if you put on 3 pounds or more, *reverse* the cycle. Or, if at any time, though your weight loss is still maintained, the cycle begins to *bore* you even in the least, *reverse* the cycle.

Once you have completed *three* cycles of diet switching, you can *rearrange* the four or five or six diets *according to your own feeling*. But if you gain 3 pounds or more, *go back to* your original cycle according to your answers to the ten questions.

And *that* is exactly how you switch . . . and achieve your normal weight.

29

When *Not* to Switch—and Other Variations

NOW THAT YOU HAVE A CLEAR SCHEDULE FOR switching the diets, let me give you a couple of examples indicating other possibilities that may be right for you to one degree or another.

One man stayed on the same diet for six months!

His answers to the ten questions indicated that he should begin on the Six-Small-Meals-A-Day Diet. He was about 25 pounds overweight. The first week, he lost 8 pounds. The second week, he lost 5 pounds. Excited by dropping almost half of his overweight, he wanted to stay on this diet. I had no objection. Within three more weeks, he was within a handful of pounds of his ideal weight. The diet, which was evidently perfect for him, was as effective as ever, and had not become a bit boring to Don. So not only did he stay on it, but when he reached his normal weight a few weeks after, he remained on the Six-Small-Meals-A-Day Diet to *maintain* that weight. And when he did switch to his second diet after six months, I must tell you that it was more for the sake of switching than anything else. "Look," I told him, "you probably should stay on this diet permanently. But just for the sake of playing it safe and refreshing yourself a little, why not switch to your next diet?"

Don did, and it worked out all right. But after ten days, he wanted to switch back. By all means, I told him. He's been on it ever since, and his weight has been within a couple of pounds of what he wants, ever since.

This *is* an extreme example, but it brings out an important point about BDS: The idea of switching is so powerful that some people hardly need to do it. You might ask, "If this man stayed on the first diet for six months and only switched once, how is this evidence that switching works? He really hasn't switched at all."

The answer is that Don's case is an extreme yet logical extension of what many people feel about the Berkowitz Diet Switch. Because they have the security of knowing there is always "some place to go," they don't have to go there!

One of the most oppressive things about trying a diet is that, in the back of your mind (and sometimes right in the front), you feel, "If I go off this diet, I have no place else to go. I'll go back to overeating." The demand of that situation—which is really the situation of every diet you've ever tried before the Diet Switch—is too big to bear. It tends to *make* you go off your diet. Once you do, it tends to batter your attitude into little pieces, so that it's even harder to get back on the diet.

Eating too much or too frequently, you see, is basically a state of chaos. You may not know where your next meal is coming from, but you sure know it's coming. The only way you can deal with it is to say to yourself, "I've got to eat less." But how? You're in limbo. And once you do get back on your diet, or don't eat as much, hanging heavy over you is the knowledge that you fell off it before, and you can fall off again.

Sensible switching removes the chaos. It always gives you a place to go. Because of that, sometimes you can stay right where you are!

The other side of this coin is illustrated by Maggie B. An extremely high-strung person, Maggie was the type of individual who seemed to have one crisis after another in both her personal life and career. The way she'd relax after meeting the latest crisis—or in the days of tension and anxiety preceding it—was to sit down to a good meal. Or snack. It would have been easy—but unproductive—for me to say to her, "Have fewer crises in your life, be a less high-strung person, and you won't have an eating problem." Life is filled with problems! And there is no island that is more attractive in the face of them than eating. Almost all of us are like this now and then. Some of us pretty consistently.

I'm no exception. There is nothing that pushes you off a diet faster than boredom or anxiety—not having enough in your life or having too much going on in it. Who among us can consistently achieve a perfect balance? Well, the BDS doesn't presume to banish life's problems magically, though it will get rid of one large anxiety—overeating and overweight. And this may help you somewhat with the rest.

Anyway, the BDS worked beautifully for Maggie, but, at the same time, it didn't work. All six diets were positive for her, and she embarked on the first, then the second, then the third, for two-week periods. After a few days on each diet, she lost several pounds. The trouble was that the final ten days of each two-week period she *didn't* lose. On a couple of her diets, in fact, she gained back some of the weight she'd lost.

I advised Maggie to cut down the two-week period to four days. Eventually, it became three days for each diet. She had hardly gotten on each diet when it was time to get off.

Forty-five pounds overweight when she began on these three-day periods, it took her only several cycles—a little over two months—to achieve the weight she wanted for the first time in seventeen years. She continued this three-day switching permanently, and has never been overweight since. Sometimes, she even switches after *two* days!

Again, Maggie and Don are extremes. But they are points along a continuum, and where you as an individual should be can be revealed only by you after your first few switches. Do *begin* with two weeks in mind. If you wonder whether it should be shorter or longer, a good rule of thumb is this: If you're less than 25 pounds overweight, you should lose about 25 percent of that overweight on each switch. If you're more than 25 pounds too heavy, it will be more like 10 percent or 15 percent. If you come close to that, fine. If you don't, and particularly if you lose more in the first week than the second, cut down on the length of most switches.

On the other hand, if at any time a particular diet—and it doesn't have to be the first time—seems to be working quite well, stay on it, extend the period from two weeks to three, four, whatever. But at the *first* sign of several days *without* a weight loss, or at the first sign of boredom, switch.

30

The Way to Weigh

HUMAN METABOLISM STILL HOLDS MANY SECRETS. one of them is why—and I'm sure you've noticed this—you can sometimes seem to overeat for a period of a day or two and not really see any effects from it. Then, suddenly, on the third or fourth day of overeating you gain tremendously.

Sometimes one large meal will seem to put on several pounds. Conversely, anyone who has ever been overweight has probably experienced this: When you're near your normal weight and you gain a few pounds, it's still easy to take them off, but once you reach a level of, say, 10 or 15 pounds above it, you have difficulty losing an ounce. Or, possibly, you have been 15 pounds overweight for some time and find that you can overeat moderately and not gain that much. Then one day you find you are gaining fast again. Once you reach another level, it's even harder to lose, though you may not gain for awhile even while overeating moderately.

Some of the metabolic reasons for this are fairly well known. In one way, the body is very much like the motor of your car. It is used to functioning at a certain level with a certain input. The difference is that your car can hold only so many gallons of gasoline and so many quarts of oil. Your body will expand to accommodate whatever you put into it. But it takes time to make the adjustment. Once you've definitely established a new level of input, the reason it's hard to take off weight is because now it is *built in*. Also, the more you weigh, the more you can eat to support that weight.

Still, as I said, there are metabolic "secrets" explaining why some of us, weighing exactly the same as someone else and cutting down the same number of calories, will lose less weight in the same amount of time. Not that the difference is ever that great over a period of a few days, but it is often great enough to discourage someone who doesn't know better.

This is why the Berkowitz Diet Switch wants to give you a couple of other ways—besides weighing—to chart your progress during each diet. Because jumping on the scale every few hours is bound to boomerang. If you find, for example, that you have dropped a fraction of a pound or more, this only sets you up to be disappointed the next time around or the time after, when you've followed the diet and the scale doesn't show it yet.

If you possess the kind of compulsion that makes you

simply have to know—and some people will weigh themselves twenty or thirty times a day—so be it. But if you can skip the scale for two or three days at a time—in fact, a weigh-in once or twice a week is enough—you may do better. For one thing, not constantly checking your weight gives you a chance to enjoy what you're eating, and to settle in on your diet. In a sense, each diet is like a new intimate friend. Or can be. Would you keep checking on your friend whom you trust and who trusts you?

Better to go by your clothes.

No doubt you have a pair of jeans, and a number of other articles of clothing, you'd like to wear but can't because they just don't quite fit. Well, give your first diet a few days, then put on that favorite skirt or pair of slacks. Still too tight? Give it a few more days. The satisfaction that comes from finally being able to fit into it—even though it's a tight fit at first—is a lot more than some tyrannical number on a scale. And by the time you switch once or twice, it will fit just fine. Then you can go on to those long-ago clothes that may no longer be in style, but will make you feel wonderful when you put them on and they fit as they used to.

Another nice way to "weigh" yourself is through photographs. Take a snapshot of yourself right before you begin on the BDS. One of your face, another of your full figure. Then take another photo when you make your first switch. And another photo with each switch. You'll love the change!

31

You Can Go Off Your Diet!

STOP.
Because you already stopped. Right?

Yes, at one time and another, you will go off even the 'diet" of the Berkowitz Diet Switch.

Fine.

Just as it was fine with Frank, June, and B. J.

Frank and his wife were invited to a small dinner party at the home of a close friend. Phil's wife had gone to great pains to prepare a sumptuous meal, beginning with the tastiest of hors d'oeuvres. Frank ate everything, including a couple of second helpings, and enjoyed every mouthful—because he *hadn't* gone off his BDS diet.

June was asked out by a junior executive of the company

where she was a secretary. Upon picking her up, Randy announced enthusiastically, "Oh, am I excited! I found this great Italian place last month. Do you like Italian food?"

Sure, June liked Italian food.

She also liked Randy.

But she happened to be on the high protein BDS diet, and the chances of eating an Italian dinner that is low in carbohydrates is about equal to the chance of teaching your pet parrot to sing the entire score of *Carmen*. Sure, she could have ordered a large antipasto and watched *him* eat. But she did exactly what she should have done—she ate a large, high-carbohydrate, high-calorie meal, and enjoyed it.

And Randy enjoyed June's enjoyment.

B. J. had been happily and steadily losing weight on her BDS diets. A graduate student at an Eastern university, she finished her reading one night and went out to the kitchen for a snack. Upon opening the refrigerator, she saw at least half a dozen things she wanted. None fit her present BDS diet.

B. J. had a piece of lemon meringue pie that one of her roommates had baked, three slices of meal loaf, a glass of wine, and two soft drinks. Which fit her current BDS diet perfectly. It would have fit *any* of her BDS diets. Because *going off* your diet is part of *staying* on the Berkowitz Diet Switch.

Other diets either want you to be a robot or want you to feel guilty when you shouldn't be. B. J's snack amounted to close to a thousand calories. She had missed dinner, which was why she was so ravenous, so she really wasn't taking in a thousand calories extra. The same goes for Frank and June. They would have eaten dinner anyway.

True, they wouldn't have eaten that large a dinner, just as B. J. wouldn't have had that large a snack. So what we're talking about here is an extra *several hundred* calories. On the one hand, that may seem like a lot. On the other, if you spread it out over three or four days, it's only a couple of hundred calories a day. By getting a little exercise, going light—not too light, just moderately—on a few meals, those extra couple of hundred calories per day are down to next to nothing.

Even if you don't cut down on a meal or two, or expend some extra calories on physical activity after you go off your diet and overeat, it's no big thing. You'd have to go off your diet not once, but *several* times, to gain even a pound.

That's why the BDS *wants* you to overeat once in a while. I'd even like you to plan for it. You'll know when the feeling is beginning to come upon you that you simply yearn to have a big meal or a huge snack. Or when you'll be in a situation that makes it impractical and thoroughly unenjoyable not to eat heartily. As long as you know what you're doing, you won't feel you're falling off the dietary edge of the earth. You'll simply say to yourself, "I've overeaten. One time. One time in two or three or four days. Big deal." You'll know it's no big deal, and you'll go right back on your diet.

Sometimes, the impulse for overeating will hit you all at once. You'll sit down to a meal, or be eating out, or be opening the refrigerator, or be passing a fast food place, and zap! Seven hundred extra calories.

That's fine, too. It's human nature for this to happen. Value it instead of panicking when it happens. Gain self-esteem from it instead of losing the handle on your diet.

For some of you it may help to jot down a couple of

times a week when you think you'll be likely to want to overeat. If it works out that way, you'll feel in control of yourself, because you'll be in control of the part of you that *isn't* in control.

If those times come along and you don't feel like overeating, don't. But some time you will. When you do, even if you didn't plan to go off your diet, remember that the plan of your diet hasn't been disturbed by nature's plan.

32

Do More—Eat More

THE BERKOWITZ DIET SWITCH DOESN'T CONTAIN ANY
exercise plans, nor does it even urge you to exercise,
though I do believe that a certain amount of regular "extra"
physical activity is almost always a plus. It's also a "plus"
in terms of the calories you can take in. The more calories
you use up, the more you can use without becoming overweight.

Here are some common physical activities, and the number of calories they burn up. I'm also including a few non-
physical activities most of us do, so that if you're sitting
around for a day, you'll know how many fewer calories to
take in:

Activity	Additional Calories Used up in 30 Minutes
Running	246
Dancing	135
Piano Playing	30
Driving a car	35
Walking fast	50
Sitting	17
Skating	128
Washing dishes	36
Eating	17
Horseback riding	51
Swimming	280
Ironing	38
Dressing	28
Carpentry	85
Sweeping	50
Typing fast	36
Bicycling	250
Mowing the lawn	245

The standard activities for most of us are sitting, standing, lying, or walking. Let's say this is more or less your daily activity: You lie down, either in sleep or in rest or in reading, ten hours a day, stand two hours, walk two hours, sit about nine-and-a-half hours, and do something a bit more vigorous for thirty minutes. It's loosely on this activity "output" scenario that most of us compute our caloric input.

But let's say that three or four times a week you dance instead of sit for half an hour. This amounts to an extra 118 calories expended. Well, you can take in that many "extra" calories.

Obviously, there are hundreds and hundreds of activities. I've given you enough of a sampling, however, so you can pretty well tell about how many calories a particular activity uses up. Of course, there is physical activity and then there is physical *activity*. Square dancing and disco dancing use up a lot more calories than swaying to music that is soft and smooth. I know one fellow who plays tennis quite well, beats most of his opponents, yet hardly ever moves off the baseline. He probably uses up only a third of the calories during an hour as his opponents, since they're racing here and there to retrieve his placements.

So don't assume that because you're involved in a certain activity, you always use up a definite amount of calories. The intensity of the activity is a big factor.

Still, though there is a wide range of varied activities, after the first couple of weeks on the BDS, you'll know whether you're counting too many or too few calories for your physical activities. Simply make the adjustment in your calculations and act—or eat—accordingly.

But don't become a "reducing bookkeeper." As long as you're within 10 percent or 15 percent of what's accurate, no problem.

Just as I don't want you to become a "reducing bookkeeper," I don't want you to become an exercise nut, either. To each his own, of course. If you really love physical activity, you should do it. Exercise can increase the utilization of calories, and improve muscle and body tone. There is good evidence that nonstop moderate exercise for thirty minutes or more can increase cardiovascular efficiency. Most of all, exercise works hand in hand with keeping your weight down by improving your self-image and your appearance.

However, physical acitivity should be based on common sense and medical knowledge. In particular, you must heed the warning signals of your own body, such as muscle pain, fatigue, or difficulty with breathing, which indicate you're approaching the limits of your physical tolerance.

Physical activity is a very individual matter. I honestly don't think some of us were made for much physical activity. For others, it's almost a necessity. In terms of the BDS, the point isn't *how much* "exercise" you get, but keying the *output* of calories expended through physical activity to the number of calories you take in. People are so tunneled in on how many calories they're eating that they often forget this most fundamental truth: If calories weren't used up by the body, you'd never lose any weight, you'd just keep gaining and gaining!

We burn up calories even while sleeping. The physiological processes of the body are a form of activity. But, obviously, simply breathing and the circulation of our blood and so forth are relatively minimal processes compared to jogging, a good game of tennis, or some vigorous work in the garden. Nevertheless, sleeping has one advantage over any other form of activity: You're sure to lose some weight while you're doing it.

So get to know your activity pattern and, based on what it is, make allowances up or down for your caloric intake, no matter what BDS diet you're on. Don't try and change your activity pattern because you're going on the BDS. I'm not pushing exercise. You don't have to jog, play tennis, or work in the garden for the Berkowitz Diet Switch to work.

33

Some Additional
Do's—and Don'ts

T IE BERKOWITZ DIET SWITCH GIVES YOU A WAY OF EAT-
ing and enjoying it, without overeating. But some of
your old habits, because of old, unworkable diets may per-
sist for awhile. Once you recognize them, they usually disappear pretty quickly. For example, a fair number of people
get into the habit of eating while they are doing something
else, just as they might light a cigarette while doing something else. Rather than eating—or smoking—for the pure
pleasure of it, they wind up smoking two or three times as
many cigarettes or eating twice as much food.

The BDS tends to eliminate this kind of behavior by encouraging the enjoyment of meals and discouraging the

denial of feeling filled. Still, if you find yourself in the habit of eating this or that without even thinking, try these two things:

1. Remove easily accessible foods from the tables in your home or office. One of the marks of a good home, supposedly, is to have nuts or candies strewn around in various bowls. But this can also strew some pounds around your waistline. It is far better to eat purposefully and at certain times than at random without really paying attention to what you're doing.

2. Identify three or four of the main "situations" in which you tend to fall into this habit of eating without thinking. And make a habit of identifying these periods, so that a STOP sign appears in your mind the next time you begin to do it.

A second habit that leads to overeating is the "leftover" habit. My coauthor had a grandmother who was never seen to eat more than one helping of anything, yet she was a hundred pounds overweight. Nor was she a secret eater. What did make her fat was the habit of not being able to carry the plates from the kitchen to the garbage can. Somewhere along that fifteen-foot route, she ate virtually all the leftovers, sometimes from half a dozen people's plates.

The "leftover" habit has mainly two roots. The first is what is often called the "economic depression mentality." People who went through hard times hate to throw anything away. So, rather than serving themselves, they get into the habit of eating very little the first time around, and filling up on what everyone else in the family leaves.

A second major reason for leftover eating is what you might call the "invisibility syndrome." What it amounts to is that some people actually feel they are eating less if no one else sees them eat, or if they are eating food that wasn't prepared for them specifically. Sure, it's silly, but you'd be surprised how many people feel that certain foods have less calories after they've been left over from dinner than at the dinner table.

Another important cause of overeating and overweight is a different kind of habit—anxiety.

As I've mentioned throughout this book, though the BDS will go a long way in many cases toward alleviating other problems you have, it is a treatment only for overweight itself. Some of us lead tense lives, and we're going to sit down to lunch or, more likely, dinner, and be tense. It would take another entire book to tell you how to switch from that tension to true relaxation.

But there is one "shortcut." I'm talking about tranquilizers, particularly before dinner.

Tranquilizers are one of the three or four most abused and overused drugs in this country. Generally, I'm against the chronic use of tranquilizers. However, for a certain percentage of people, a mild tranquilizer taken an hour or two before a meal can make a world of difference in whether or not you overeat. It's fine for someone to tell you, "Simply relax and take your time eating," but most of us don't have that much time most of the time. And you can't relax by pushing a button. If you *can* schedule your dinner a little later or your lunch in a more relaxed situation, eating much as you do in a fine restaurant, one course at a time, taking your time, wonderful.

Yet for all but a few of us that would be the exception rather than the rule. So what you need is something to cut through the tension *before* the meal so that you will relax during it, savor your food, eat enough but not too much, and come away with a feeling of self-esteem.

However, there are tranquilizers and there are *tranquilizers*. One doesn't have to take a pill to take the edge off the tension and truly enjoy dinner without gorging. Some people like to have a drink or two before the eveing meal. Alcohol in moderation, drinking slowly to allow time to feel its beneficial effect, to relate to someone else, or even to watch TV with a glass in your hand before eating, will probably do you more good than harm. There was a study not long ago that showed moderate drinkers seem to have a longer life expectancy than those who don't drink alcohol at all. However, drinking too much is worse than not drinking at all. So, the before-dinner drink or two must be for the purpose of feeling good and enjoying the meal, not a habit that applies to other times of the day.

Some people find sex a tonic before dinner. It's difficult if you have kids who are eagerly awaiting the call "soup's on!" But for the many couples for whom children aren't a problem, a little love-making now and then before the evening meal can be a marvelous tonic. You're relaxed afterward, and you're eating much later—which makes a large midnight snack unlikely. Last but not least, the pleasure you had through love-making makes the need for pleasure at the dinner table a little less urgent. At the same time, you've had two or three or four hours of "uninterrupted enjoyment," and after a hard day, you deserve it!

There are a variety of other tranquilizers available to you.

Some people like to exercise before dinner. I don't. But if you can handle it, and you don't have to rush it, it can work in your favor, very much like love-making.

Keep in mind that "after" is almost as important as the "before." If you are rushing *from* a meal, you lose the savor of it. Schedule an extra half-hour—even ten minutes—after each meal for simply digesting it.

Needless to say, if the "tranquilizer" you take occasionally before a meal is in pill form, you should consult your doctor. Don't buy some over-the-counter pill.

However, the best preparation of all for meals while you're on the BDS is these two things: (1) learning to value that "hungry" feeling, and (2) eating a full meal—or a full snack.

When someone says an athlete has "that lean and hungry look," they mean that all other things being equal, he or she has more desire to win. By the same token, a *hungry feeling* before meals helps to make for a lean person.

Remember when you were a kid and you'd get so taken with playing you'd forget to eat? When it finally got dark, and it was time to come in, you were famished and loved just about everything your mother put in front of you, including second and third helpings. And you didn't get heavy. The kids of today don't know this feeling quite as much, partly because of TV. But it's a healthy feeling, and it's one you should cultivate again as an adult.

Almost unknowingly, you see, we Americans have been propagandized against the most natural, healthy feeling in the world—hunger. We've almost been made to be afraid to be hungry!

This propaganda comes at us from many directions. The

media hammers away with ads about this food or that. Manufacturers spend millions packaging products attractively, and supermarkets line the shelves with them, so that it is almost impossible to walk in without buying several items on impulse. Restaurants want you to eat out. Fast food chains want you to drive up. Even the government gets in on the act, for, as people spend more on necessities, it gives a lift to our sagging economy.

So growing up in an America where food, food, food seems to be surrounding you everywhere, it's little wonder that by the time you become an adult, you feel it's almost unhealthy or a sign of failure not to have a full stomach constantly. Earlier, we talked about the "depression mentality," which causes people to carry a few extra pounds or even a potbelly because they were traumatized by living through a time when food wasn't plentiful. Younger generations, though they haven't lived through the depression, have become so inured to "the good life" that they frequently fill up on five- or six-course meals and seldom know a true feeling of hunger when the next mealtime comes around. The youngest generation of all, kids who sit in front of the TV, are the worst victims. Sure, they get some exercise now and then, but few of them have ever known genuine hunger enough in their life to remember it as a *real feeling*. They, like too many of the rest of us, go by the *taste* of food, not the *inner need* for it. And when you do this, you tend to move more toward overweight. If you're hungry, a huge lettuce and tomato salad tastes wonderful. If you're full, the taste of a salad pales next to a candy bar or a pizza, or a dinner at a fine restaurant.

I'm not against dinners at fine restaurants. I love to eat

out now and then at a special place. But those who do this continually often find that the fine restaurants begin to taste alike. They start looking for new and more exotic places. Their tongues become jaded, and their waistline widens.

Stop to think about *hunger* for a moment.

What's the parallel to hunger in other realms of our existence? Sexual lust and passion for one's partner is one, isn't it? Certainly that's a good thing. Ambition in our work, which is the keynote to accomplishment and self-esteem, is another. So *why* do we put down hunger?

The Berkowitz Diet Switch is probably the most permissive and individualized reducing plan imaginable. Yet don't use that freedom to lose the wonderful, vigorous feeling of hunger that is natural to any animal. Now and then, when you do become hungry on your BDS diets, *stay hungry* for a while. Or simply skip a meal now and then so that you can know real hunger and enjoy the next meal ten times as much.

I know, grandma always told you not to miss a meal. And grandma was right for *her* time. But that time was when food was not plentiful, when we were not an affluent society, when the majority of our population was not overweight, and when most of us did physical labor during the greater part of the day.

Cultivate that hungry feeling. And you'll cultivate that lean look.

And once you've cultivated that hungry feeling, make sure you satisfy your hunger.

Not only does the BDS want you to eat what you like, but just as important, to come away from the table *feeling satisfied.*

By far the main reason for the habit of overeating, over-snacking, eating without sometimes even knowing it, and most other diet problems *is that we don't satisfy ourselves at meals.* We want to lose weight, so we skip breakfast and are so hungry by midmorning we consume high carbohydrate snacks or too much for lunch and dinner. Or we sit down to lunch, "discipline" ourselves by eating something low in calories that doesn't really satisfy us, then gorge ourselves at midafternoon, dinner, or later on. And so it goes.

And the overweight doesn't vanish away like that.

With the Berkowitz Diet Switch you come away from each meal feeling happy and satisfied because you choose what you like best to eat from each type of diet. In the beginning, of course, your metabolism and your somewhat "stretched" stomach will be used to more food, and this is why we have diets allowing you to eat more actual food and take in less calories. Because you enjoyed your last meal, you will look forward to your next one.

After a short time, days probably, you will have even stronger motivation to wait for that next full—but not fattening—meal. The motivation will spring from the fact that you have lost pounds. After a few weeks, you'll have lost a truly meaningful number of pounds, but your motivation will lessen. The diet you are on will begin to lose its newness, its excitement. There are other foods in other diets that you won't have had for awhile. You'll begin to long for them. If you were on some type of diet other than the BDS, you would then begin to "go off" your diet, and it would begin to fail.

But with the Berkowitz Diet Switch, the next step is precisely to "go off" your diet and onto another you've been waiting for.

And then again. And again. You can see why the BDS works.

Most people who have tried the Berkowitz Diet Switch say that its main asset, the "wonder" of it (as one woman who went from 173 pounds down to 128 within a few months expressed it) is that *you look forward to eating.* And not only your next meal, but your next *diet.*

Of course, as a man who succeeded on the BDS once asked me afterward, "Suppose I had simply taken this food or two from this first diet of yours, this one from another, these from another, this one from another, made sure they balanced nutritionally, and added up the right number of calories from each. Wouldn't I have lost just as much weight?"

The answer, I told him, was yes. But I added, "What you're talking about is an ideal way of eating—which indeed 3 or 4 percent of us are naturally capable of. But if you had *done* that, if you could *do* that, you never would have been overweight in the first place!"

I know *I'm* not a perfect eater. If I depended upon eating *only* a balanced diet that was *just right* in calories for me, *day* after *day, year* after *year,* I'd be a lot *heavier* than I am now. I would go through periods of depriving myself, when I would either end up overeating, or take out my lack of food fulfillment in some other part of my life and create for myself even larger problems.

And speaking of problems—

Though I sincerely feel that the BDS *can* be, in the figurative sense, a "panacea" for those of us who are overweight, it is, of course, no panacea for life's problems in general. Is *anything?*

Still, there *is* a relationship between problems and

pounds. When we are suffering from anxiety, or depressed and unaware of it, we tend to eat more. Sexual difficulties, when not confronted, often channel themselves into over-eating. Financial pressures may make us fat. Subconsciously, a full stomach or even a potbelly can subliminally signify the security of knowing we can go without the next meal, that we have something "in the bank." And so on.

Again, the BDS doesn't purport to solve your financial, sexual, or any other problems. However, you'll be happily surprised to know that the majority of those who have been able to achieve an ideal weight and pretty much an ideal way of eating by the BDS frequently experience a dramatic improvement in other areas. One of the reasons is obvious: We are *whole beings,* and if we can get a handle on one of our major problems, we have that much more time and energy and confidence to deal with the others.

But there is another good reason. Solving one major problem—especially that of overweight—can give us a *model* and *method* for dealing with the rest. It is important to know the inexorable fact that *you are bound to experience improvement in other areas whenever you conquer one.*

In 1979 I counseled a married couple, both of whom were overweight. Both suffered psychosomatic medical symptoms, from headaches to fatigue. This was partly because they were high-strung people. It was partly because they had chronic anxiety due to a couple of continuing problems. One was that their sexual relationship wasn't what it could have been. The other was that they were overweight. We are *disturbed* by excess poundage. It gives us anxiety. Depresses us. Lose the poundage, and you lose at least *that* anxiety and depression.

After a few months they could see that the BDS was working. Their sexual relationship began to improve!

After a few more months they were reasonably certain that the BDS was the answer to their overweight. The man was within a few pounds of his ideal weight, and his wife was *at* her ideal weight. They also confided to me that their love-making was now idyllic!

I'm not telling you that so dramatic an improvement is inevitable in that short a time in *every* case. But I will tell you this: *If you understand that SOME improvement in other areas of your life is virtually inevitable, you may experience tremendous "fringe" benefits from the BDS.* Self-improvement is, to a great extent, a self-fulfilling prophecy.

34

An Adventure . . .

AND NOW YOU ARE READY TO EMBARK UPON A GREAT adventure—a whole new, permanent way of eating what you prefer, as pounds pare away, self-destructive eating habits disappear, and unworkable reducing regimens become unnecessary.

Yet since you haven't actually experienced it, I want to assure you that, most of all, the BDS won't take anything away from you.

Know that.

You can have your favorite foods, and because you're having them, you won't need to overindulge yourself. Now and then, you will, because you're human. And the BDS allows for that too.

Food is wonderful. Eating is wonderful. I want you to enjoy the foods you love, I want you to look forward to eating—and to know that the BDS is built upon this.

Once again, the Berkowitz Diet Switch won't take anything away from you.

Except pounds.

Excess pounds.

Please understand that you don't have to struggle to do it. Dieting doesn't have to be a battle.

Stop struggling.

Stop fighting.

Switch.

APPENDIX A

Weight Charts

WOMEN

Height	Ectomorphic Build	Mesomorphic Build	Endomorphic Build
5-1 to 5-2	101-109	106-118	114-130
5-2 to 5-3	103-111	109-121	117-132
5-3 to 5-4	107-115	112-124	119-137
5-4 to 5-5	109-118	115-128	123-140
5-5 to 5-6	112-121	118-133	127-144
5-6 to 5-7	116-125	122-137	131-147
5-7 to 5-8	121-129	126-141	136-153
5-8 to 5-9	125-133	130-145	139-156
5-9 to 5-10	128-138	134-149	143-160
5-10 to 5-11	132-142	138-153	147-166
5-11 to 6-0	136-146	142-157	151-171
6-0 to 6-1	141-151	146-162	156-175
6-1 to 6-2	145-155	151-167	160-180
6-2 to 6-3	150-163	155-172	165-184

(Weight Charts Continued)

MEN

Height	Ectomorphic Build	Mesomorphic Build	Endomorphic Build
5-3 to 5-4	117-125	122-135	131-146
5-4 to 5-5	120-128	126-137	133-150
5-5 to 5-6	122-131	128-141	137-154
5-6 to 5-7	126-134	132-145	141-159
5-7 to 5-8	130-139	136-151	146-163
5-8 to 5-9	134-143	140-154	149-168
5-9 to 5-10	138-147	144-158	153-172
5-10 to 5-11	142-152	148-163	157-177
5-11 to 6-0	146-156	152-168	162-181
6-0 to 6-1	149-161	156-173	166-187
6-1 to 6-2	154-165	160-177	170-192
6-2 to 6-3	158-169	164-182	175-197
6-3 to 6-4	162-173	170-187	180-202
6-4 to 6-5	166-178	175-191	185-207
6-5 to 6-6	171-183	179-195	190-212
6-6 to 6-7	176-187	184-200	195-218

APPENDIX B

Calorie Charts

Approximate Calories in Common Alcoholic Beverages

	Calories
Ale (1 bottle)	190
Beer (1 bottle)	148
Light Beer (1 bottle)	85
Brandy (2 oz. glass)	162
Champagne (3 oz. glass)	90
Eggnog (1 cup)	250

Cocktails:

Daiquiri (4 oz. glass)	110
Manhattan (4 oz. glass)	90
Martini (4 oz. glass)	86
Tom Collins (6 oz. glass)	124
Whiskey Sour (6 oz. glass)	130

Mixed drinks containing:	*Calories*
Gin (2 oz.)	192
Rum (2 oz.)	236
Bourbon (2 oz.)	123
Rye (2 oz.)	123
Scotch (2 oz.)	108

Wines:	
Dry (2 oz. glass)	92
Sweet (2 oz. glass)	162

Approximate Calorie Counts of Common Beverages

	Calories
Apple juice (1 cup)	120
Carbonated beverages (cola-type, 1 glass)	105
Chocolate milk (1 cup)	190
Cider (1 cup)	122
Coffee, black	0
Coffee, with sugar or cream (1 cup)	98
Ginger ale (1 cup)	83
Grape juice (1 glass)	118
Malted milk with ice cream (1 large glass)	500
Milk:	
Buttermilk, cultured (1 glass)	85
Skim (1 glass)	87
Whole (1 glass)	164
Orange juice, frozen concentrate (6 oz. can)	304
Orange juice, fresh or canned, unsweetened (1 glass)	118
Prune juice, canned (1 glass)	173
Root beer (1 small glass)	47
Tea, unsweetened	0
Tomato juice, canned (1 glass)	48
Vegetable juice (1 glass)	39

Approximate Daily Caloric Needs For Average Somewhat Active Adults

WOMEN

Height	Ectomorphic	Mesomorphic	Endomorphic
Not quite 5'	1900	1950	2015
5' 0"	1960	2010	2075
5' 1"	2020	2070	2135
5' 2"	2080	2130	2195
5' 3"	2140	2190	2255
5' 4"	2200	2250	2315
5' 5"	2260	2310	2375
5' 6"	2320	2370	2435
5' 7"	2380	2430	2495
5' 8"	2440	2490	2555
5' 9"	2500	2550	2615
5' 10"	2560	2610	2675
5' 11"	2620	2670	2735
6' 0"	2680	2730	2795
6' 1"	2740	2790	2855
Taller than 6' 1" but not taller than 6' 3"	2800	2850	2915

Caloric Needs For Average Adults

MEN

Height	Ectomorphic	Mesomorphic	Endomorphic
Not quite 5' 3"	2300	2350	2415
5' 3"	2360	2410	2475
5' 4"	2420	2470	2535
5' 5"	2480	2530	2595
5' 6"	2540	2590	2655
5' 7"	2600	2650	2715
5' 8"	2660	2710	2775
5' 9"	2720	2770	2835
5' 10"	2780	2830	2895
5' 11"	2840	2890	2955
6' 0"	2900	2950	3015
6' 1"	2960	3010	3075
6' 2"	3020	3070	3135
6' 3"	3080	3130	3195
6' 4"	3140	3190	3255
Taller than 6' 4" but not taller than 6' 5"	3200	3250	3315

APPENDIX C

Composition of Most Common Foods Used on the Berkowitz Diet Switch

Food	Amount	Carbohydrates (Grams)	Protein (Grams)	Fat (Grams)
Apple	1 average	21	Almost none	Almost none
Apple Cider	6 fl. oz.	20	Almost none	Almost none
Applesauce, unsweetened	½ cup	12½	1	Almost none
Apricot, fresh	1 cup	21	1	Almost none
Asparagus	1 cup	17	3	Almost none
Avocado	½ cup	4½	3	19
Banana	1 average	27	1	Almost none
Barley	¼ cups	40	4	Almost none
Beans, green	½ cup	4	1	Almost none
Beans, kidney	½ cup	21	16	1
Beans, lima	½ cup	18	17	1
Beef	4 oz.	0	45	9½
Beets	½ cup	6½	1	Almost none
Blackberries	4 oz.	13½	1	Almost none

Blueberries	½ cup	10½	1	Almost none
Bread, cracked wheat	8 oz. slice	11½	2	1
Bread, whole wheat	8 oz. slice	10½	3	1
Broccoli	½ cup	4	3	Almost none
Brussels sprouts	½ cup	5½	4	Almost none
Butter	1 tsp.	1	Almost none	11½
Cabbage	½ cup	3	6½	Almost none
Cantaloupe	½ avg. melon	13½	1	Almost none
Carrots	½ cup	4½	1	Almost none
Cauliflower	½ cup	2	2	Almost none
Celery	1 oz.	1	Almost none	Almost none
Cheese (all kinds)	1 oz.	1	5½	8½
Cottage cheese	1 cup	5½	34	9½
Cherries, sweet	½ cup	11½	2	Almost none
Chicken	4 oz.	0	21	3
Corn	1 cup	27	3	1
Crab	4 oz.	1	16	2
Cream	1 cup	10½	7½	29
Cucumber	1 avg.	6½	1	Almost none
Dandelion greens	½ cup	5½	2	Almost none
Dates	1 cup	135	4	1
Eggs	1	.4	5½	5½
Endive	1 cup	3	4	Almost none
Escarole	1 cup	3	4	Almost none
Fish	4 oz.	0	16	4½
Flour, buckwheat	1 oz.	21	1	2 Almost none

Food	Amount	Carbohydrates (Grams)	Protein (Grams)	Fat (Grams)
Flour, corn	1 oz.	22	2	1
Flour, whole wheat	1 oz.	21	2	1
Frankfurter	1	6½	6½	16
Fruit, cocktail, unsweetened or dietetic	½ cup	7½	1	Almost none
Gelatin, dietetic	½ cup	0	5½	Almost none
Grapes	½ cup	6½	1	1
Grape juice, unsweetened	4 oz.	18	1	Almost none
Grapefruit	½ avg.	13½	1	Almost none
Grapefruit juice, unsweetened	½ cup	11½	1	Almost none
Ham	1 oz.	0	19	20
Honey	1 tsp.	18	Almost none	0
Kale	½ cup	2	2	1
Lamb	4 oz.	0	44	11½
Lemon juice	1 tsp.	1	Almost none	Almost none
Lettuce	1 cup	2	1	Almost none
Lime juice	1 tsp.	1	Almost none	Almost none
Liver	4 oz.	5	32	11½
Margarine	4 oz.	.5	1	48
Mayonnaise	1 tsp.	.3	Almost none	10½
Milk	1 cup	11½	8½	8½
Muffin, corn	1	21	3	4

Food	Serving			
Mushrooms	½ cup	1	4½	Almost none
Mustard greens	1 cup	8½	3	1
Noodles	1 cup	39	6½	2
Oatmeal	1 cup	27	4½	2
Oil, salad or cooking	1 tsp.	4½	0	13½
Okra	½ cup	4½	2	Almost none
Olives	1 avg.	.1	Almost none	Almost none
Onions	1 avg.	8½	2	Almost none
Oranges	1 avg.	20	1	Almost none
Orange juice	½ cup	12½	2	1
Oysters	13-19 avg.	7½	21	4
Papaya	1 cup	19	1	Almost none
Peas	½ cup	9½	5	1
Pea soup	1 cup	23	8½	3
Peach	1 avg.	9½	1	Almost none
Peanuts	½ cup	12½	19	38
Peanut butter	1 tsp.	3	4	7½
Pear	1 avg.	26	1	1
Pecans	½ cup	7½	4½	40
Peppers	1 avg.	3	1	Almost none
Pineapples	½ cup	10½	1	Almost none
Popcorn	1 cup	7½	1	Almost none
Pork	4 oz.	0	47	22
Potato	1 avg.	22	3	1
Potato chips	10	9½	1	7½
Raisins	½ cup	57	2	Almost none

Food	Amount	Carbohydrates (Grams)	Protein (Grams)	Fat (Grams)
Raspberries	½ cup	9½	1	1
Rhubarb	½ cup	2	1	Almost none
Rice, brown	4 oz.	30	4	Almost none
Salad dressing	1 tsp.	1-4	Almost none	4½
Sauerkraut	1 cup	5½	2	Almost none
Spinach	1 cup	1	4½	1
Strawberries	1 cup	11½	1	1
Sweet potato	1 avg.	38	2	1
Tangerine	1 avg.	9½	1	Almost none
Tomato	1 avg.	6½	2	Almost none
Tomato juice	½ cup	4½	1	Almost none
Turkey	4 oz.	0	21	3
Turnip greens	½ cup	3	3	Almost none
Veal	4 oz.	0	24	13½
Walnuts	½ cup	8½	14	40
Watermelon	1 cup	9½	1	Almost none
Whitefish	4 oz.	0	16	4½
Wine	3 fl. oz.	1-22	Almost none	Almost none
Yams	4 oz.	28	2	Almost none
Yeast	1 oz.	3	3	Almost none
Yogurt, plain	8 oz.	12½	7½	4
Yogurt, flavored	8 oz.	45-55	6½	7½

Index